Why Do You Call Me Mom?

The Experience of an Alzheimer's Patient's Caregiver

Linda Marie Hoffman

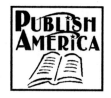

PublishAmerica
Baltimore

First printing

PublishAmerica has allowed this work to remain exactly as the author intended, verbatim, without editorial input.

ISBN: 1-60672-931-4
PUBLISHED BY PUBLISHAMERICA, LLLP
www.publishamerica.com
Baltimore

Printed in the United States of America

Acknowledgments

First and foremost I thank my husband, Rod, who made it possible for me to write this book mostly because of his full support and deep commitment in helping me to care for my mother. Also to the many other family members who helped in the care of my mother along with the encouragement they gave me to not give up. To my two sons, Rich and Tim, and daughter Shalene, who were my life support and they continued to encourage me to write this book. And to Molly, my niece, who was forever faithful in caring for her grandmother. To mom, the most loved mother in the world, who opened our eyes to the disease called Alzheimer's.

Contents

Introduction

My husband and I were, as far as we knew, set in a comfortable lifestyle. We worked along side each other in a family business of 24 plus years. With three children and ten grandchildren, we had a full schedule of baseball, basketball, football games and dance recitals on our calendar. I also was involved with my charity work at the church. We had vacations planned a year in advance with our grandchildren. We thought our lives wouldn't change.

However, all of this was turned upside down in just one short week, when we made the decision to care for my mother. My work schedule changed from eight hours, five days a week to four hours for four days a week. There would be no more church volunteer work, seeing my grandchildren's games or dance recitals, or planned vacations. My mother had Alzheimer's disease and needed constant attention on our part.

Alzheimer's disease takes a toll on the patient and everyone around the patient. It's hard to watch people slowly lose their memory and ask questions, such as "Why do you call me mother?" Questions that show patients don't know who their caregivers are can be hurtful and hard to handle, especially if the caregivers are loved ones. These questions put stress on the caregivers and make them not want to continue. However, continue they must. The only other option for family members is to put their loved ones in a nursing home, which might not be able to take on such patients, depending on the type of facility.

Patients with Alzheimer's disease don't start out that way, however. They don't immediately forget their children's names or how many they have. It's a slow process over time. In the beginning, patients just ask caregivers to repeat answers to questions that were asked five minutes, or fewer, prior. This can get aggravating to have someone continually ask the same question, over and over again.

The problem with this disease, or dementia, or any that involves losing memories is that caregivers don't forget, just the patients. Caregivers endure a lot of stress over many years and usually have no outlet for their stress or pain. Many times, the caregivers are alone and have no one to help with taking care of the patient so they get no time to themselves.

I dealt with my mother's Alzheimer's, and the stress associated with it, by writing in a journal. This book is the result of that journal. I want to give information and inspiration to fellow caregivers dealing with similar events. But, most of all, I want caregivers to know they aren't alone and that many others feel the same as they do, even if they can't express it.

Chapter 1
Period of Adjustment

In the beginning of caring for a patient, family and friends need time to adjust to a new routine and having a new person in the house. Adding new people to any household would require homeowners to change their routines to accommodate these new people. This is true for parents giving birth, parents adopting a child, those caring for elderly relatives or those having relatives visit for a period of time. Caring for sick relatives presents additional challenges on top of those involving daily routines. However, Alzheimer's patients present unique challenges beyond those of ordinary sick relatives that caregivers probably won't begin to realize. After a few weeks, the routines are set, and the challenges are overcome with solutions. Although, this doesn't necessarily mean it will become any easier.

Floating Banana Peels

The first week my mother lived with us was quite interesting and a learning experience for all of us – me, my husband and sadly for my grandchildren who lived down the street, and regularly came to visit us.

I remember the second day especially well. We found banana peels floating in our swimming pool. I had no idea why they were there. I found out later that my mother threw them out there. All

my large cooking pots from my kitchen were filled with water and
placed in corners of the back yard and in the kitchen. We realized
from these two incidents that we had to always watch what my
mother did and keep a continual eye on her.

The Food

On the fifth day, I was ironing with my country music playing.
I was enjoying myself because my mother was in the next room
sleeping or so I thought. My granddaughter came in the house and
asked why there was stuff on the lawn and why the back door was
propped open. I realized my mother had awaken, quietly went
into the kitchen, and propped the refrigerator door open with a
chair. She took all the food out and set it on the counter and
outside on the lawn. Because of this incident, I got angry with my
mother.

I said, "Mom, what are you doing with the food? You're going
to ruin it."

She looked at me and said, "I don't know who this food
belongs to, but it doesn't belong to me so I'm getting it out of my
kitchen."

I had yelled back that this was my kitchen and to put the food
back. The biggest problem came when her dog tore open the
package of bacon and had eaten all the leftover fried chicken.
The dog also got into plastic containers, making all the food
inedible. My husband heard the yelling and, after looking at the
kitchen and yard, took my mother for a walk while I cleaned up
the mess with my granddaughter's help. I was mad. Our emotions
didn't mend as fast as I cleaned up the mess. I had to learn how
to deal with my initial shock and emotions. My mother didn't
understand the yelling or that she lived in my house. I learned that
I had to lighten up a bit if this new life was going to work for all

of us. I started calling it our house, which allowed my mother to let go of her shield and anger.

Mom and Her Dog

In addition, with the other incidents occurring in the beginning of the week, I felt helpless and angry. My mother had a unique relationship with her dog. She wanted me to feed it constantly, and she thought people were stealing it when they were only taking her for a walk. We had to adjust to issues with the dog, as well.

For example, one day, while sitting at the kitchen table paying bills, I looked up and saw my mother coming down the hall fully dressed with her brown purse hanging off her shoulder. She said, "I'm ready when you have time to take me home." I tried to reason with her. I told her she was home. She felt sad and betrayed. I learned to change the subject quickly when it came to issues that made her sad but that took time to learn. I would say, "Can we go to the store first?" She usually went to the store with me or to a fast-food restaurant for a cheeseburger.

On that particular day, we went to a restaurant with her dog and mine. We loaded the dogs into the car. We bought cheeseburgers for ourselves and the two dogs. Her memory never failed when it came to her dog. She never forgot the name of the dog and wondered who would take care of it when she was gone. She also assumed my dog was hers and told me to feed it so it would grow. She couldn't understand why the poodle was small. I wondered why Alzheimer's patients can remember information about certain things, such as their pets and nothing else. Research should be conducted on this phenomenon.

Eventually, my mother no longer asked about going home after these trips. She believed that she was home where her dog was. She commented to me one time, long ago, that she knew she was home if her husband was around her. Now, she felt that way about her dog.

Toward the end, she forgot the dog several times. She would ask, "Whose pretty dog is that?" We would answer, "Yours." She said, "I'll take the dog if no one else will give him a good home. He can live with me." We stopped saying "your dog" because she would worry about feeding it and having money to care for it. We would eventually start answering, "Our dog" or "The dog lives here."

The Last Party

My mother also hurt my grandchildren's feelings on the night after moving into our home. She didn't recognize them, despite loving them and knowing them the previous year. She accused them of stealing food from her and her money.

In caring for my parents, I have undergone many changes in my life even regarding mundane things. I have three married children and 10 wonderful grandchildren. Some of the grandchildren have steady girlfriends or boyfriends. All these people came to Sunday dinner once-a-month or used to come.

That all changed when I started caring for my mother and father. I had to spend more time with them, especially with doctor visits in that last year before my father died. Many times, my father would call me and tell me he didn't feel good or tell me my mother hadn't gotten out of her chair all day. My husband and I would drive over to my parents' house. I never knew whether I would be gone for a half hour or four hours.

Things started to change long before my mother moved in the house with us. I spent less time with my family and less time at my job. The gatherings with my children became fewer and fewer because I never knew when I would get called away. We still got together for birthdays and every few months.

After my father died and my mother moved into our home, we couldn't get together for birthday parties any more. She couldn't handle large groups of people or the noise. If there were more than two people in the room talking at a time, it confused her, making her nervous and angry. All these people talking, that she didn't remember scared her. She didn't know what they were saying or who they were. She would start shaking and tell everyone to go home while pointing a finger right into their faces. I was especially upset when she scared my grandchildren.

When I hadn't seen my grandchildren for 10 months, I decided to have them to my house for Sunday brunch. My husband said he would try to keep my mother occupied with the dog inside the house while we ate outside the house. All morning, as I made cinnamon rolls and cooked, my mother stood in the kitchen looking at the food. She leaned against the counter. My husband and I were ready at any moment prepared for what might happen next. I was hoping she wouldn't argue with me over whose kitchen, stove and pots and pans I was using. My mother always believed the kitchen was hers and no one else's. No one was allowed in it.

All was well. It was the largest meal I had cooked in a long time. Cooking had always been my passion, a trait I inherited from my mother. She was a wonderful cook before the disease claimed her life and we always appreciated that part of my mother. She went out of her way to cook for others.

As each family member came, they were careful not to be too loud. We put the small children outside the house. The adults got to enjoy their meal inside the house. Everyone talked in a whisper. My mother sat in her chair with her dog beside her, looking out the window, while sipping iced tea. My teenage granddaughter came in the house at this time. She had been late because she had to work that day. As she filled her plate, my mother walked into the kitchen and looked at everyone at the table. She yelled, "Who is cleaning up this kitchen?" She was so angry and yelled at everyone. Each member of my family stood up to leave. But my mother yelled some more, "Who decided to have a party in my house and invite all these people that I don't know?" Everyone stood in silence.

Everyone pointed to me, but no one said a word. My granddaughter put her plate down untouched and said, "I'm outta here." I grabbed her arm and said, "No, you're not. Sit down. No one is going anywhere." I told everyone to eat and have fun. My granddaughter said, "Oh great. Now we have two insane women in the kitchen," as she sat down with my hand still on her shoulder.

However, I was no match for my mother. She stood firm as she pointed to all the dishes and food. She continued her rant about cleaning up the mess. My son-in-law stood up and told my mother that he was in charge of cleaning the mess. We all laughed as he told everyone to leave and pointed at me to clean up the kitchen. He thought he could calm her down or at least make her laugh.

Unfortunately, the laughter backfired. My son-in-law was trying to help me, but my mother got angrier because she no longer could understand what he said or why it was making everyone laugh.

I spent the next 45 minutes giving my mother really sweet iced tea that she loves. My daughter-in-law, whom my mother thought was a 12-year-old school friend, helped me calm down my mother. Everyone moved to the back yard with food still in their hands, and they tried to keep quiet. She remembered that they went outside with food. The rest of the day, my mother repeated that strangers were in her house and took her food. She was worried she would starve. All of us were sad that we made her think such thoughts.

An hour later, my husband sat on the sofa next to her. He put warm blankets from the dryer on her legs because she was shaking. I never knew if the shaking was from nerves or a chill. For two hours, they sat there. She kept asking my husband to tell her who they were that took her food. My husband said he told them to leave and not come back. Late that night, my mother finally forgot about the strangers.

My daughter-in-law and I wondered as we cleaned the kitchen why some things are forgotten in seconds and others linger for hours. We wanted her to forget about all of her "food being taken". We didn't want her to go to bed with that thought.

I fixed her a plate of fruit that she ate. She asked if we had anything for breakfast. I told her we had some food in the kitchen, so she was satisfied enough to go to sleep. We stayed with her until she changed her thoughts from starving to believing we had lots of food in the kitchen. My daughter-in-law helped me get her in her gown that evening as we repeated over and over about going to the grocery store for food.

The blessing of that day was that I was able to go to a part of the yard unseen from the kitchen or family room and spend time with my children. My grandchildren were upset that day, but they understood their great grandmother was ill. We told them she had Alzheimer's disease. It took some explaining, but they began to comprehend.

What to Do?

My husband and I took these incidents into account when we discussed my mother that first week. We weren't sure we could handle these kinds of situations that would occur as we dealt with caring for my mother. We both worked outside the home and would have to rearrange our schedules to accommodate my mother. However, I considered that someone who didn't love my mother could take advantage of her so we agreed to adjust to our new lives.

Home

Home became an issue with my mother. It was one I had to deal with carefully. Learning the right words to say was difficult at first but became easier as time progressed.

On this particular day, my mother came to me and asked, "Is there any where I can wash my hair in this place?" I answered yes even though she just washed her hair at 2 p.m. the day before.

She then said, "I don't know who you are but this is a really good place to live. You have lots of room here. Are any for rent? Can I sleep here tonight?"

I realized my mother had a new definition of home. Her definition wasn't what ours would be. To her, home meant a roof over her head and a clean bed, but it's not a place where she could connect with other people whom she loves. It's a structure to keep her safe.

I said to her, "Yes. There is a room here, just for you as a matter of fact. Would you like to go back and look at it?" Her yes indicated that she was more grateful for a roof over her head to protect her from the darkness outside than for the love I offered her. The comment didn't offend me, but it did make me sad. I loved my mother and wanted to take care of her, but she didn't know that any more. I wasn't her daughter. I was an innkeeper. She never knew my goal and purpose in life now was to care for her.

My mother would pack pillow cases with her purple gown, underwear, several T-shirts and framed pictures of people she knew. Some of them weren't in our family. Sometimes, she would get angry because she didn't know where her husband was because she had her bag packed and was ready to go home. We would sit at the kitchen table and discuss my father and why he wasn't with her. I would say he was working and went fishing. I used his name when we discussed him. After a while, she would look at the pillowcases and wonder who put them in the kitchen. Then we would look for treasures in the pillowcases. She would take out everything and then put everything back into the pillowcases. It would keep her occupied. But there were times that she would recognize her things and think I was going to steal them from her. This happened after we got my mother back to her bedroom and I put them away. I reassured her that her clothes were safe and were where she put them. She would say, "You don't know who lives by you. We have to be careful." It made me sad that she thought I would steal from her.

All day, my mother would walk from one end of the house to the other talking about where she would sleep. At night, her ankles were swollen and blue. Even after she got on her gown and we hoped the pacing was over, she wouldn't stop. My husband would watch television in the family room until 11 p.m., that night, to make sure he could see whether she wandered, and she did continue to wander until the wee hours of the morning. I stayed awake and kept watch so I could let him go to bed.

A Fright at Night

After my mother finished her breakfast, my mother asked if we had a bathroom. She couldn't remember where it was or that she had gone 45 minutes earlier. I had a hard time being cheerful and happy. She had slept late and was well rested. She was in a happy state of mind so I had to be and do everything in my power to keep her that way.

However, while my mother was well rested, I wasn't. I woke at one o'clock in the morning to have my mother looking down at me in my bed. It frightened me. I screamed, which woke my husband too. It took me two and half hours to get her back to her bed. She insisted I was sleeping in her bed. After discussing this over and over, my husband told me to forget it because I wouldn't win. But I knew that if I waited another 10 minutes, she would forget what we were arguing over and I could get her back to bed. And, about 10 minutes later as I sat on the edge of my bed while she stood at the dresser, she asked, "Why were we in the dark?"

I learned to use "therapeutic fibs" in situations like these. I told her that she wanted to use the bathroom, and then I directed her back to her bed. My mother began shaking. She was scared and frightened. That night as I sat on her bed talking, hoping she would fall asleep soon, she tried to get up several times. She was scared. Finally, I lied across the foot of the bed and fell asleep. I knew she would disturb me if she tried to get up again. After several hours, I went back to my bed.

My husband asked if I got my mother settled, but he wasn't as worried about the incident as I was. She was truly frightened, and not knowing if she would sleep until morning or get up again concerned me. She could fall, or worse, she would be afraid in the dark unless she found me.

This was one of the many times my mother was frightened at night. Just as night was a frightening time for my mother, it became something I dreaded, as well. I never knew how my mother would respond each evening when the sun went down, or late into the night. All precautions were taken to start reassuring her early in the evening. We hoped we would eliminate anything that would make her think about the night.

Often, we would start by saying, "Aren't we lucky to have an inside bathroom now." Or "All the animals are fed and down for the night so we have nothing to worry about." She often worried about going outside at night to use an outhouse, not remembering inside bathrooms. It was strange that my mother never forgot we had an inside bathroom during the day. Only at night did she think we had no plumbing and had to use an outhouse.

However, trying to keep one step ahead of her thoughts didn't start early for me. It was a learning process, but I soon learned it quickly.

The Problem with Stove Knobs

I was in the shower after I put my mother to bed fairly early one evening. She wasn't afraid or didn't ask too many questions that night about my father. When my husband came into the bedroom, he whispered, "Better hurry up and get in the kitchen. It's getting bad." A hundred thoughts went through my mind. She still often surprised us. I washed off the soap as fast as I could and put on my robe. It would have been such a pleasure for me to take a long shower and not be in a hurry because I knew my mother was already asleep.

My mother had all the food out of the refrigerator on the counter, had two burners with two pans on them and nothing inside them. She had left over chicken and meat loaf in pans or plates on the floor feeding both dogs. Her dog would eat all night long if she was given the opportunity. My mother was enjoying this. She put meat into her hand to warm it by squeezing her hands together and then put it in the pans on the floor. She looked at me and said, "I think that man who stays here is mad at me, but I had to tell him if he didn't like the way I feed my dogs, he could just leave my house."

I listened to her say it several times hoping she wouldn't get any angrier at my husband because he had tried to stop her. He soon found out that there was no stopping my mother. I had learned to talk her out of situations, but my husband couldn't talk her out of something without making her angry. After 30 minutes, I got her to wash her hands and change gowns. She had food all over herself, and then I put her to bed again. I put all the meat in a bag for the dogs for later, cleaned all the bowls and pans off the floor. My husband took the burnt pans outside the house. We had to hide the stove knobs that night where they stayed for the next year. My mother and I had many more arguments over the knobs. The hiding of the knobs was a necessary step to protect my mother and ourselves.

I walked back to my mother's room to see if she was still asleep. She was sitting up in bed and asked if she had fed the dogs yet. It was hard for me not to scream yes at her, but I had to be patient and remember that my mother had forgotten everything that happened.

Later, was when my husband and I discussed taking off the knobs. He felt so bad about having to get me from the shower. But he also realized the mess and smell wouldn't have been so bad if the knobs were gone. He was upset he couldn't talk to my mother and reason with her. He was just a man that lived in the house, not a son-in-law to her.

On another Saturday morning, my husband said he would stay inside the house with my mother so I could do yard work and plant flowers. It had been a week since I had stepped outside the house.

At about 10:00, my husband opened the kitchen window and said, "You are needed in the kitchen." I frowned. When the kitchen is mentioned, it is never a good thing. I asked if my husband could handle the situation a little longer. I was almost done with my yard work. He told me to come now. I walked into the kitchen with dirt and potting soil on my hands, to find my mother had put a new roast, already cooked that we haven't eaten, in a pot of water to boil. She also had taken a frozen roast from the freezer and put it in another pan of boiling water. It still had the plastic wrapper on it.

I lost control and asked my mother what she was doing with the chicken she held in her hand. I said the chicken was already cooked and had paid $8 for that cooked chicken, for tonight's dinner. Most of the chicken was torn apart and boiling over in another pan. It smelled dreadful. My mother got upset from my yelling and from calling her mom. She said, "Mom, mom. I don't know who you are but stay out of my business and my kitchen. Alfred will be home soon and he'll be hungry."

It took me a few minutes to adjust. Water was boiling everywhere. I needed to calm down to handle this situation and get her out of my kitchen. I turned off the burners and told my mother the meat was done. I asked her if I could help her clean up the kitchen and by the time we got her cleaned, she had forgotten why she was mad and why she was in the kitchen. However, she remained mad the rest of the day. I was frustrated with my husband, who I thought was watching her, while I worked in the yard. He had fallen asleep watching television.

I have learned that most of these issues can be resolved without showing emotions. We took off the knobs for the day, but we should have left them off the stove permanently. Anger and embarrassment are the two biggest outward symptoms of Alzheimer's, which are visible daily, in patients. When patients can't remember something, they get embarrassed. They then get angry. However, they can't remember *why* they are angry, which makes them frustrated. I also became frustrated with my mother and myself. It only made matters worse when I showed how mad or frustrated I was. I had to learn to not show my emotions. As soon as I calmed down and lowered my voice, I was able to get to focus on cleaning up the kitchen and getting her away from the stove.

Home-Care Aids

Two aids were able to last quite a long time caring for my mother. There were others, but they couldn't handle my mother. When my father took care of my mother, several aids left before they got in the front door of their first visit. Before the ones that did stay most of the two-year period, we did have many that lasted only a few days, especially after they found out my mother had Alzheimer's. None of them were experienced to care for Alzheimer's patients. We were blessed with those two that did stay throughout the two-year period my mother lived with us.

Before she came to live with us, though, the agency would call my father or me and tell us that my mother ran them off with a fly swatter, hot cup of coffee, or held the door shut telling the caregivers they were at the wrong address. My father never said anything. He didn't want to get her into an argumentative mood, knowing it would last for days.

When we had exhausted all available aids from one agency, we called another and said I would be there at 8:00 a.m. when the aid arrived. Still, none would be able to stay more than an hour. Several mornings, my sister and I took turns being there at 8:00 a.m. for the new aid and would let her in the house. We would sit on the front porch. My mother would come out and sit with us, thinking the aid was our friend. My mother still wouldn't let her help with breakfast. She would tell the aids, "Go home and eat. Why do you want to eat in my kitchen? Don't you have a home of your own?" Then, she would lock the door. I couldn't even get into the house myself, at times. At the time, my father was so ill. I thought he was just tired from my mother pacing all night. I could have helped him more if I had known then what he was going through. I now know.

The problem was that strangers weren't welcome in her house. This was different from my childhood when my mother would cook and feed the whole neighborhood. She would also give food to the poor. That's when I decided that this wasn't my mother doing these things to these aids. We are who we are by our actions and deeds; whether evil or kind, not by our physical bodies that we were given. My mother's body hadn't changed, but her mind had. I had to learn to deal with this new creature in my mother's body. This was a whole new mind set.

My hope is that researchers will create a medicine to slow or stop the progress of Alzheimer's. At any point during the care of my mother, I would have been thrilled to have a medicine that could keep Alzheimer's from getting worse and keep the brain standing still. But she didn't get any medicine like that. We did try a new medication for three months, but my mother got progressively worse. My father ordered her off the medicine. I didn't know why, but we all agreed to take her off because her insurance didn't pay for the drug, anyway. She did seem to be worse.

After my father died, we had eight aids total. Two only stayed for one month. My niece got certified during those two months and became a real lifesaver. At first, my mother occasionally remembered her, but after three months didn't. My mother became more difficult to handle. My niece started to take all the angry words and moody spells personally. After six months, my niece met me as I got out my car and told me she couldn't help me with Grandma any more. She normally has the patience of Job, and is very kind. She told me she didn't know how I could do it every day for seven days a week. She said she was here only four hours a day and couldn't handle it. She took it upon herself to call the agency to send someone new next week. This news made me freeze. My niece had been faithful, not missing a day. If she did, she made up the hours so I could work at our construction office.

My mother had told her she wasn't her granddaughter and to get out of the house. She told my niece that she was mean to her. If she were related, she would take her home where she belonged. She told my niece she came over to the rental home and to eat all her food. My mother was afraid she was going to starve. She asked her if that is how she's supposed to treat a grandmother. My niece felt betrayed every time she saw her grandmother. She felt angry about the Alzheimer's disease and told me she couldn't do a good job any more.

Her husband told me later that my niece would come home every afternoon crying, sometimes up to three hours. I wasn't aware what was happening, because I was too busy attending to my mother in the afternoon that I couldn't spend time talking to her on the phone. We would leave messages for each other by tablet or by phone what we both needed to know about my mother for that day. We couldn't talk because my mother was usually sitting or standing next to us and if we mentioned her name she got mad or embarrassed. My mother always would say when two people talked, "You are talking about me. I know it." Then she would start yelling at us.

The second long-term aid finished out the assignment. She did quit once after a year. She needed some rest mentally from the stress of Alzheimer's care. We talked her into coming back after five weeks off, going through four aids, none of whom returned after more than three days. Cindy loved my mother and I can't repay her enough for the good care and love she showed her under the most difficult and exhausting circumstances. It was amazing how she knew when to back off if my mother became angry and how she instantly could show love five minutes after my mother accused her of stealing everything in the house, of kidnapping her, or leaving her to starve in the house where she knew no one. Cindy always said, "I tried to place myself in her shoes. How can I get mad at Ruby? She is so lost." Cindy tried hard to make my mother feel safe. She said that was her job and she took it seriously. I used to say that Cindy was a Godsend.

We did the best we could to make my mother's last months comfortable.

Scaring the Aid

The day didn't start out good at all if my mother woke up angry. I knew she probably would stay that way all day. She wouldn't eat before I left for work. She was giving the aid mean looks. The aid called me at work and asked me to come home. She had tried to give my mother vanilla pudding and she pushed it away yelling at the aid. I got two hours of work done. The aid told me my mother had told her that she was giving her someone else's food and told her to call the person who lives at the house. My mother locked herself in her room and wouldn't leave.

When I got home, I told the aid to go outside the house for a while or into another bedroom. I needed to calm my mother down. She was angry and wanted the aid to leave the house. My mother didn't think the house was safe with strangers in it. She felt that people kept coming in and out the house and bothering

27

her. My mother repeated this mantra over and over. She started pacing back and forth, which scared me. I was afraid she would fall. Her balance wasn't good at that time. She also was getting weaker all the time because she didn't eat much.

My mother yelled and pointed a finger at her. She even tried to push the aid. Despite my efforts, nothing seemed to calm my mother. I let her yell for a while and then tried to change the subject. I asked her if she fed her dog. I usually didn't mention the dog, but this time, it worked.

The aid left for the day, which meant she didn't get paid. Although I felt bad about that, I knew it was the right thing to do. My mother needed someone to blame that day for her confusion. That was the aid. When these incidents happened later, I worked out a program with the aid to have her do other things away from my mother so she could get paid. She was able to help me during those times. The aid was a trooper to deal with my mother's rants for four hours. But those four hours seemed like an eternity to the aid at the time.

Walking the Dog

My mother always thought someone was trying to steal her dog. My husband and I were the only ones she would let walk the dog. Sometimes, she let my grandchildren walk the dog.

In the beginning, a friend would come over and take my mother's dog for a walk. When my father died, my mother would smile when our friend came. The dog would go crazy, bark and stand by the leash at the back door. This routine only lasted a few months. It became such a strain on us.

At first, my mother would say, "Oh here comes that girl who walks my dog. No one else will do that for me. She's the only one in this whole world who will help me with my dog." We all did, but my mother couldn't remember.

After a few months, when our friend rang the bell, my mother would tell me not to answer the door because there was a woman trying to steal the dog. I was frustrated. Here was someone who wanted to help and do us a favor, but my mother wouldn't let me answer the door. I tried to explain that my friend just wanted to take the dog for a walk, but then, my mother would get outraged and told me I was working with my friend to steal the dog. She went to her room and locked her door. We let her stay in there while my friend walked the dog. By the time, my mother had left her room, she had forgotten what had happened. But those visits from our friend stopped after a while. I couldn't talk to her for a year. When we saw each other again, we didn't mention the dog.

The Back Door

The day after Christmas, my son-in-law came into the kitchen to cut a piece of chocolate cake. I was on the back porch when I heard a loud scream. I came running in the house to find my mother yelling at him and trying to take away the plate in his hand. He stood frozen. He's 6 feet tall and weighs 250 pounds, but he was scared of his little grandmother-in-law. I had to laugh. He was truly hurt as she yelled at him to get out of this house. She was mad that he was stealing food from a poor woman. She started worrying about starving to death. He backed out the door as I grabbed my mother who was shaking again. She couldn't walk. I later took cake out to him. It was months before he came back into my kitchen. Even though people who are around an Alzheimer's patient understand these reactions, they still get hurt feelings.

Almost an hour later, my daughter-in-law came into the kitchen to get a sugar cookie. My mother jumped from her gold chair. She asked whether my daughter-in-law only came over to eat. She smiled and told my mother she was the best cook in town. My daughter-in-law always could get her to calm down. My mother smiled back and said it took three or four hours to clean up the kitchen and not to make it messy again. She ran out the back door with a handful of cookies. My mother sat down and resumed her cold stare into space.

My children got used to using the back door or just staying in the back yard if they wanted to come visit me. If they went to the front door, the dogs would bark and she would know they were here. I never knew the reaction they would get from my mother, and neither did they. It was easier to stay in the back.

My son often told everyone, "Better go to the back door and call Mom on the phone first unless you want to take the chance of having Grandma yell at you or accuse you of stealing from a poor woman."

Shoe Hide-and-Seek

One particular morning, my mother sat at the kitchen table eating and being very quiet, and was in deep thought about something. She drank her coffee and as I unloaded the dishwasher, I made sure that she saw me. I kept busy in the same room where she sat. If she couldn't see me, she would go back and forth looking for me, saying "You are the one that I know helps me." I also wanted to make sure that she finished her cereal.

She looked up from her bowl and held her spoon. She asked me if my husband was dead. She asked that same question yesterday at the same time. I told her he wasn't dead and would be home soon so she could see him. She said she hadn't seen him

30

in years and that it would be good to see him. Right before taking another bite, she said she had some boys that I know are dead. I told her she had boys. I knew I had to change the subject. I asked her if she wanted any toast. She said she would if I ate some toast also.

My mother went back to her room to get dressed. I had laid out her clothes beforehand. She looked at the clothes and wondered where her shoes were. I told her she wore them when she ate breakfast. She said she hadn't eaten breakfast and hadn't left her room. I knew the day wasn't starting out well. She hid the shoes. This was the beginning of what would happen for six months. We found them after 20 minutes searching her room. They were in an old heavy plastic overnight bag full of books in the back of the closet.

This hunt for shoes would prepare me for the next several months of shoe hide-and-seek. It became a common practice of getting up at night and hiding them. After three weeks, I started putting a pair of slip-on sneakers in my closet when I went to bed at night. That way, I shortened my hunt for the shoes the next day. She never left her bed without first putting on her shoes. If she couldn't find them quickly, she would yell about her shoes.

Later, she put all her shoes in a pillow case and carried them around everywhere. She hid each pair several times. I was so tired. I finally told her to look for the shoes herself. She looked disappointed at me and said, "You're standing there with shoes on your feet and have plenty of shoes in your closet. I have none. You don't ever care about an old woman barefoot." It was certain she had more energy than I did that day.

I laughed about the incident with my husband that first night. After the next several nights, it wasn't as funny any more until we put the pair of shoes in my closet, for safe keeping. Most of the time, she would look for the shoes herself and sometimes, it was hard to get that one pair from her room at night for me to hide. On a few occasions when I got back into the room thinking she was asleep to sneak the shoes out, there would be my mother. I knew we would be going on the hunting trip early the next morning.

No More Church

I took my mother to church two Sundays after she came to live with us. On the first Sunday, she was so excited, but when it was time to leave, she sat down and decided she didn't want to go. She couldn't remember if she knew anyone there. I got very upset because I had gotten all dressed, and it took a very long time to get her into the shower that morning, get her to eat and get her to wear her best clothes.

She put on black pants after my coaching. I told her to wear pants to church now because she didn't have a dress that fit properly. I also changed from my dress into pants so she would feel better about wearing pants to church. That meant I changed clothes twice myself.

Finally, I got her into the car and we were on our way. I just knew that when we got there, she would love it. My father hadn't taken her to church in two years or more. We sat toward the back, which ended up being a good idea because as the music started she got very upset because it was so loud. I could tell she was getting nervous and frightened. It was hard to get her to speak softly when she was asking questions about the service. We finally got up and left early. I had to help her out by holding onto her arm and guiding her to the door by almost pulling her at times. My mother was distracted by all the people and microphones. It became overwhelming for her.

We skipped the next Sunday, but by the third Sunday, I thought we would try it again. This time, it was easier getting ready. I put pants on her and myself. As we were leaving, she sat down in the kitchen chair and said, "My feet hurt. Do I have another pair of shoes?" I got her another pair of dress shoes and knelt down to put them on her feet when she pulled both her legs under the chair and said, "I don't know whose shoes those are, but they aren't mine. Those are men's shoes." I tried to talk her into them, but it didn't work so I got another pair of shoes, which she wore. We were off to church.

This time, we sat in the very back row, and my daughter also sat there with us. As the music got loud, my mother started to shake and get upset. We talked about leaving, but my daughter said, "Just wait a few more minutes." After that amount of time had passed, everyone had stood and shook hands with each other. My mother wanted to know why the man in the front of us had shorts on, I tried to explain it, but it wasn't working. Then another couple came in and that man also had shorts on. My mother got so upset and started talking very loudly about the men in shorts. My daughter said, "I think it's OK Mom if you need to take Grandma home now." We left. I told her I had to go to the bathroom. We never went back to church. It was funny that she remembered people were supposed to dress their best for church, but she forgot to talk in a whisper or what she was there to do.

Chapter 2
Moving Away from Denial

Alzheimer's patients forget the world around them, but the family never forgets. When a patient is diagnosed, the family goes through a period of denial. They usually want everything to be the way it was, but it can't be. At times, I denied what happened to my mother. Other times, my siblings thought my mother would be all right with some prompting. My children and grandchildren couldn't understand why their grandmother and great-grandmother said mean things or hurt them. They wanted to put the blame on the disease, but, in the moment, remembering the changes in their grandmother was difficult. I found, though, that the sooner the caregivers and their family moved from denial, the easier the job of taking care of patients became.

The First Time I Knew

I first heard someone suggest my mother had Alzheimer's disease while I was visiting my parents' home. A next door neighbor and I were talking over the fence. She said, "Your dad told me Ruby has Alzheimer's disease." I froze at the news. I didn't hear anything else she said after that even though I politely let her finish her conversation. Later, I asked my father about it. He said, "You know your mom is very forgetful and confused a lot. That's how her sister got when she had Alzheimer's," which was my aunt in Chicago.

I couldn't accept my father's diagnosis because my mother ate healthy foods, exercised on the tread mill, rode a bicycle, walked every evening after dinner, and never went to a doctor. I couldn't see how someone so healthy could have Alzheimer's because she was never sick. I mean never!

One day, I called her. She told me my father was mean to her. She was crying. After a while, she calmed down when I told her I would be up to see her the next morning. My parents lived four hours away from me. I made the trip every other Friday to go check on them before we moved them closer to us. I called her again, later in the day. She was upset but she couldn't remember why. I talked to my father. He had been gone all day and said he was going to bed now because he was tired. He told me that he would talk to me in the morning when I got there. I thought of them all night long. I was worried.

When I got there, I asked my father what had happened. We had to go outside the house to talk because he said my mother would get mad at him. He also said the utility company called to say they were going to turn off the electricity. He asked my mother about whether she paid the electric bill. She took care of all the finances. My father then said that they had went through the checkbook. When she couldn't see where she wrote out the check, he yelled at her. He told me that he had said, "If you wrote out the check, you should remember." I found this odd. My father never yelled at my mother. That's why my mother broke down. He took the checkbook to the utility company and paid for the last three months of bills for water and electricity that were unpaid. That was the reason he was gone all day. He had to get all the bills figured out. He felt so bad about yelling at my mother, but he was unable to calm her. That's when I called on the phone.

Oddly, I was so glad it happened, because I knew they needed help.

Later that day, my mother asked me to look at her bills. From that day forward, my sister and I took turns writing out the bills and balancing her checkbook. After that day, I looked up every piece of information on Alzheimer's disease and called the support's help line. Unfortunately, no one could inform me on what was to come. No information could prepare me for caring for my mother. I wasn't around my aunt at all when she had the disease so I didn't have a clue what she experienced, except that my cousin said my aunt was just plain mean and should be placed in a nursing home, and she was.

I wished there were a book that encouraged caregivers not to give up and not take anything to heart that a loved one says, with the disease. I wanted a book to tell me not to get my feelings hurt, and to enter the world of the patient and leave mine behind. I also needed to know to nod and agree even if I knew I was right and my mother was wrong. All these things keep balance and puts peace and calmness in the household, which is especially important for the patient. My mother's thoughts weren't rational. I had to remind myself when she would talk fondly of my two oldest brothers, that she couldn't remember her other five children and that it wasn't her fault. I also reminded myself that she was talking to her sister and not her daughter. My mother thought I was her baby sister most of the time.

Some doctors tell caregivers to be direct and to not lie. I found this to be impractical advice. During the care of my mother, I found if I had to say no to end a situation, that I always knew I had to stick around to face the consequences. I couldn't let my emotions run wild. Alzheimer's patients aren't themselves.

Till Death Do Us Part

When we moved my mother and father to live closer to us, we were concerned for my father whose health was failing. He needed help caring for my mother, who often forgot things. At the time, we thought she forgot things because of age. We later found out that it was Alzheimer's disease.

I often wondered how my mother could have Alzheimer's. My mother was healthy. She was mobile. However, her forgetful mind interrupted my parents' life style.

Even though my father had just turned 87 and my mother 85, we thought that my mother would be the one to die first. She always told him, "Well Alfred, I sure hope I go before you do because living alone without you would be unbearable." My father always answered, "Oh Mommy (his nickname for her), chances are we'll go home at the same time together." She would smile.

In some ways, it was as he said. Taking care of my mother took a toll on my father. When he passed away in early September, my mother was in the same room, but she really wasn't there. She never comprehended what had happened. Even if she did know what had happened, she understood only for a few moments before forgetting again.

For the next 18 months, I would relive my father's death every single day. If I told her my father died, she would scream this horrible cry and asked me for proof. I would show her the pamphlet from the service or show her the guest book from the funeral home. She also yelled at me that I would keep this from her and keep her from missing the funeral. Keeping this information from her wasn't human, she said. An hour later, my mother would ask all over again where Alfred was. I would go through the ritual again. I would cry, not because of Dad, but because of that scream that I can still hear today. My mother's sadness made me sick, as I cried with my mother, finding out for the first time that her husband was gone and having to relive this day over and over.

Finally, enough was enough, I had said, as I talked with my niece who said she couldn't take the crying and reliving her grandfather's death. I called the doctor and asked her if there was any reason we couldn't tell my mother that my father had just gone fishing. I thought the tears would stop then. We did do that. It made all our lives easier but I didn't grieve my father's death until after my mother died. I was too busy taking care of her that I didn't have time to miss him. Now I miss both of them.

Dad—A Forbidden Word

My mother stayed in her room almost the whole day this Saturday. This was only the second time she remained in her room. She got dressed in the evening. I said nothing because I didn't want to embarrass her.

Throughout the day, I went into her room. She would be sitting on her sofa, counting her money in her wallet. She would look at me and try to hide the money. Later, she would tell me to come to her. She would say she had money. That knowledge made her happy.

She also walked down the hall to the entryway of the kitchen, but she would walk back to her room. I brought her a sandwich, but she was too busy counting her money to eat. I left it there with her favorite drink. A half hour later, my mother had eaten half of the sandwich.

Before dinner, my mother got dressed and thought she had been dressed all day. I could see she was tired from walking down the hall so much and eating so very little. I helped her brush her teeth two times and got her ready for bed. She asked whether she would get her things back. I pointed to different items in the room and explained that they were her things. I showed her the trunk she had when she first married my father.

She asked about him. I told her he died. She started crying loudly. She was upset about her father, not mine, and also her sister. I tried so hard to change the subject but she only talked about her father. She told me about the time she and her sister worked in the field so hard when they were young and how unhappy they were. She cried over her father's death like a little girl and this time, I didn't know what to do.

We gave her a sleeping pill but even at 10 p.m., she still talked about how hard they worked and how her father was gone. She was so scared. Her eyes were closed, but tears were coming down her face. I sat on the side of the bed late into the night to ensure she was asleep. I hoped she would have a better dream than reliving a bad childhood memory.

We had decided that we couldn't let her go to sleep that sad and unhappy again. We decided that we could move her to a different part of the house where the memories wouldn't be. We would try to get her on a different subject.

I believe that her childhood must have been full of sadness and hard work, but she never talked about it to her children. Her life was full after marriage, with seven children, social work, and church volunteering.

This experience also taught me not to use the word, "Dad," as this made her think about her father. When I referred to my father after that, I called him Alfred. That way, I didn't trigger memories of her past childhood.

My mother's legs were swollen from shoe hunting and her feet ached this day. I rubbed them with lotion and pain cream. She had no idea why her feet hurt so much. I knew why mine hurt! Shoe hunting takes a toll on your feet and back.

She sat on her sofa after getting ready for bed, hoping she wouldn't get up because her feet and legs were red. I told her to stay there with her feet raised. She said she would stay if that would help her feet. I told her it would. I got pillows and made her comfortable. I turned on the television and smiled. She said Alfred used to cut her toenails. I said I remembered Dad cutting her toenails. Looking down at mine, I told her that my husband wouldn't cut mine.

She looked at me, staring again. She wondered whom I meant by "Dad". I had to think about what I had said. I told her Alfred was my father and her husband of 68 years. She said nothing. For a long time, she stared. After a while, she asked if I meant William P. Cox. I told her Alfred was my father, but she got angry and sat straight on the sofa.

My mother talked about moving to this town and how hard it was to make a living. In her world, I was her baby sister. My mother talked about things and the hard life they had farming. I realized she must have had a difficult and sad childhood. Later, I called my aunt and questioned her about these things. My mother never talked about her childhood when I was growing up. If it were one she wanted to forget, the disease would bring back the memories and force her to live through it again.

The conversation upset her a lot. She didn't close her eyes before midnight. My lesson from this experience and a previous one was that her mind would wander to her childhood or her family whenever I said "Dad". That evening I told my husband that we must think before saying "Dad" or it would trigger old memories. This had happened several nights in a row.

The Upside of the Disease

Every time my mother started her afternoon ritual of pacing and worrying about where she would stay that night, I would worry that she would wander outside the house looking for someone familiar or something for herself. In this state, she could have let the dog out the door that would run away. I also feared that she would wander away herself.

I found out that some Alzheimer's patients recognize that the day is about to end. It's called "sundowners." But they can't recognize a kitchen or room at night that they knew in the day time. This was hard for me. I worried about what she would do in this state. My husband and I had to keep our eyes on her until she fell asleep during this time.

The upside of the disease came from a doctor who made the latest house visit. She told me not to worry about my mother wandering. She told me my mother wouldn't wander far and, after a few months, she wouldn't venture outside the house any more or get into a car. I asked for doctor visits once-a-month to help me adjust to being a care giver. The one time I could vent was when the doctor came every month. That truly came to be the only time I could say anything, and it became a time of venting for me. No matter what I said, it wasn't strange to the doctor. She had heard it all before me. When we talked, she didn't look at me like I had two heads!

It was nice to be allowed to speak and not be judged that I was either "exaggerating," as my family often said, or not doing a good enough job caring for her. I stopped talking to them because of it. The doctor often said she would tell me when she thought it was too much for me to handle. She did at the end, about three months before my mother died. The doctor encouraged me all along and even near the end when we told her we wouldn't put my mother in a home. The doctor made phone calls to me more often and stayed in touch with hospice. It took so many people to care for one person, I found out.

It also helped that my mother never knew she had Alzheimer's disease. My father didn't want to tell her. Even when we were discussing her illness with her sitting next to us, she didn't understand that we were talking about her. She would look at us and nod as if we were discussing the man next door.

This wasn't the case in the beginning, but as the disease worsened and the doctor or a hospice worker came to check on my mother, we would talk. My mother thought we were talking of someone else. We never said her name.

First Christmas

After my father died, my mother constantly asked me where her man was. On the first Christmas after his death, my mother knew that things had to be done, but she couldn't remember what. She knew she should be busy doing something because I was busy. It frustrated her to have to ask me what her job was.

On that first Christmas, my 16-year-old granddaughter came over on Christmas Eve to vacuum and dust while I cooked, preparing for Christmas dinner. I told her not to mention Christmas was the next day because her great-grandmother would think she had to cook. She wouldn't remember how and get angry because people were coming over to eat all her food. I have heard that so many times before this day. I no longer got upset by it. I got sad because my mother was the "queen" in the kitchen. Now she worried about starving.

My granddaughter stayed away from my mother and also avoided putting food in her mouth because she was afraid Grandma would see her. She was told to leave within 30 minutes.

She managed to get all the vacuuming done and a few other things when my mother asked her to go to her own home.

Alzheimer's is a hard disease to understand, when someone is only 16 and doing something good for someone, as she was doing. I was upset when my mother took my granddaughter's drink from her hand and slammed it on the counter and chased her out the door. I ran after her crying. She said, "I know. I know. My real great-grandma doesn't live in her body any more." No words could comfort this 16-year-old doing a Christmas deed. I was worried about the next day. I was wondering how it would turn out or how long it would take my mother to run everyone off.

My sister had called and asked me about Christmas day. None of my family had been to my house for a few months so they didn't know how much worse the disease had gotten. She said they would only have six people at their house so my mother could come there for Christmas, while we would have more than 22 if everyone came as planned.

We decided my mother would go to my sister's house. They would get her around 9 a.m. My children would come here at 11 a.m., open their gifts, have dinner and leave my home by 3 p.m. My sister would bring my mother back after 3 p.m. We thought it was a good plan.

The first thing that went wrong was my mother didn't wake up on Christmas morning. Even though I had so much to do, I kept checking to see if she was awake. She had been so excited the night before when she was in bed. We talked about the next day. She said she knew it was Sunday. She said she didn't have anything to wear to church.

I told her it was Sunday, but it also was Christmas. She got worried about not having any presents. She said she needed to buy presents for her boys. I said she didn't have to worry about presents. I told her a story. I said she had four boys and it was their turn to give presents to her.

She looked at me, not moving, with a cold stare. Again, she asked me why I called her "Mom." I swallowed, still not prepared for that question once again. I told her she was my mother. I was Linda. I told her we lived here in the house together. I said it slowly. She smiled and hugged me over and over. She wondered what she would do without me. Again, I told her "her boys" would bring her Christmas gifts. She accepted the idea and became like an excited child waiting for Santa Claus. It was after midnight when she finally fell asleep. She had no anger or sadness. I went to bed sad because that night all I could think was her expression when she asked why I called her "Mom." She said she only had boys, no daughters.

The next day was a different story. I had the feeling deep down that I should have tried to deal with my mother staying with me on Christmas Day. I hadn't seen much of my own children and grandchildren. I figured one day wouldn't hurt. My mother would be with my sister and in good hands.

I got her dressed in a hurry because it already was 9. I had to wake her. She had no cereal when the door bell was ringing. My sister was rushing. No. 1 rule: Never rush an Alzheimer's patient. I wanted my mother to open her gift from us and get a picture, but we had no time. She was rushed out the door looking mad at me, saying she didn't want to go. She pleaded with me to let her stay here. My husband helped me get her into the car with her dog. She hung onto him and wouldn't let go. I stood at the door crying as I could see her looking at me from the car. My mother began shaking all over. I didn't know what to do. My sister and my mother drove off. I had a sick feeling in my stomach, had to reapply my makeup, and wasn't ready for 22 people who would be arriving soon. I worried about her all day.

My sister called from her car at 2 p.m. She needed help with my mother who was shaking so badly she couldn't walk. Fear had set into her bones. I knew what fear can do to her. My sister didn't because she wasn't around her much. She thought that my mother just wanted to come home and that if she kept her at her house long enough, my mother would adjust, but my mother didn't. My niece told my sister to take my mother home because she wasn't having fun and she didn't know anyone.

Christmas was over for me when they arrived. My daughter cleaned up the kitchen and put away the food while I stayed back in my mother's room holding her with my husband wrapping blankets around her. I tried anything to get her to stop shaking. I called the doctor who came over the next day. The doctor said that even though she was with her family on Christmas Day, she really wasn't because she couldn't remember them. They were strangers to her. She needed to see the same faces and be in the same place as much as possible. I found out that no changes in routines are best.

When the doctor came, my mother was tired and angry. She put her arms across her bedroom door and spread her feet out against the door blocking the doctor. The doctor said my mother was fine physically as we sat in the kitchen talking. She told me that things were going to get worse, not better and asked if I could handle it. I told her I could.

My memory of Christmases will always be with me, but her memory won't. This incident made her more afraid to leave the house. I only wish my sister would have brought her home earlier, but she didn't know. Staying home was the safest place for her in body and mind. This day would have been better had my sister recognized my mother's disease. Instead, she thought my mother would remember Christmas when she was surrounded by family.

The fact that my mother couldn't remember her family was a hard concept for all of us to accept.

The Last Drive

After that Christmas, my mother only went out with me a few other times. We went to my sister's house once, but we were there for only10 minutes. My mother wouldn't sit down. She stood the whole time and asked me when we were going to leave the restaurant. She had thought my sister's house was a place to eat. Of course, my sister wanted us to stay and was upset when we left. I never thought about her feelings when we left. My concern was getting my mother home because she was upset and angry.

Driving back to our house, my mother said she didn't recognize the places we passed. She asked if I was taking her home. I told her the city had grown, and new houses were built. I wanted to get her mind off the place or home she had in her mind. I always thought that she could visualize her old home from a few years before. I was afraid she would react when we drove up to mine that was different from the one in her mind. I was afraid she wouldn't leave the car. My mother was a strong woman. I would have needed help to get her out the car. The last year of her life, she never got into a car again.

Hamburgers

It became more and more difficult to find someone to help sit with my mother when I had to run errands. One Saturday, there was a funeral my husband and I had to attend, because it was a dear friend. So my daughter-in-law said she would bring my granddaughter to stay one hour then. My daughter-in-law would be at the house the rest of the time. My granddaughter was young and might need reinforcement.

When they first got to the house, my mother was upset because my granddaughter took the dog for a walk first so she could be in the house the whole time with her great-grandma. She knew how important it was to keep a constant eye on great-grandma. But my mother got mad right away because she thought people came to steal the dog. To get her mind off the dog, I talked about the man in our front yard who was mowing. It distracted her.

My daughter-in-law brought two hamburgers and two drinks in the kitchen while the dog went on his walk. We said good-bye and rushed off to the service, and my daughter-in-law left. My granddaughter took out the hamburgers and put them on the table to eat with the drinks beside them. My mother took the hamburgers from her hand and told her she took her hamburger. She pointed to the one on the table and told her, "That one's yours, Grandma." My mother said it was for the boy who was mowing the lawn. She walked to the door and hollered to the yard man to get his hamburger and drink. My granddaughter didn't have anything to eat. She didn't want to upset my mother so she said nothing more about food. The yard man enjoyed lunch, thanks to my mother.

When we got home, my daughter-in-law was at the house and told us the story. They stopped on the way home so my granddaughter could eat. My mother kept telling us how this girl came to take her food. She kept watch and wouldn't let her have any. She had forgotten she gave her food to the yard man.

My granddaughter told us that when we left, she was "stealing the dog" and when we returned, she was "stealing the food." It hurt her feelings. She understood partially. She wondered if her great-grandma had enough to eat when she was young. She asked if her great-grandma was selfish about who got to eat. I told my granddaughter that my mother was unselfish and would go without if she thought anyone wouldn't have enough food. I tried to explain about Alzheimer's, but my granddaughter had trouble understanding.

Siblings' Denial

It became apparent that my brothers and sisters couldn't care for my mother for even two hours. I never asked for more than two hours, but it was impossible for them, anyhow. They couldn't understand why she did what she did and say what she said. I realized that I shouldn't try to understand. I told them to pretend they never saw my mother before they came. They couldn't. They always left mad at my mother, unable to pretend, or they left crying.

Two hours was too long for them. I would get angry with them, taking it way too personally. I thought they didn't want to help me, but that wasn't the reason at all. I see now that they couldn't handle the situation and stress.

Sadly, the last year, only one of my brothers came around at all. He lived out of town, about four hours away. He would come in the house and sometimes, my mother would remember him, and sometimes she didn't. At first, he thought my mother was pretending and wanting attention. He would go outside for awhile and come back in. She would hug him and say she was glad he came to visit. After he went to the bathroom or went outside and returned, she would go through the "Hi.-How-are-you?-So-glad-you-came-to-visit-me" ritual. He soon realized she had no memory. It took him months to get used to it. He cried at times, but he did come every six weeks to see her. Before she died, she didn't always recognize him, but because he was with her for either half a day or two days, every six weeks, it didn't bother him as much as the other siblings.

My point is that not everyone can handle the pressure level of an Alzheimer's patient, especially family members. I also think education is a big part of it. I told my siblings to read or talk to people about Alzheimer's and learn about the disease. That doesn't always work, however, when the patient is a mother.

The Need For 15-Minute Checks

I had to get over my mother not knowing me because she lived with me, but my brothers and sisters didn't. It tore their hearts out, I could see that now. As they would leave sad and crying, saying she was so mean, I now think that not remembering someone makes people old and mean. We are all guilty as we forget people in our lives at times.

The first time my sister came over to sit with my mother, while my husband and I went to a company Christmas party, was an eye opener for her. We had installed a television monitor in our kitchen so I could get ready for work early before the nurse came on weekdays. I could see my mother if she went into the kitchen at 6 in the morning before I could get dressed and into the living room.

My sister thought it was awful to have a camera in the kitchen spying on my mother. It also had a voice monitor on it so we could hear my mother shuffling or the dog tags jingling that alerted me that my mother was up and I needed to be where she was.

When we got home from our party, we could hear some noise coming from my mother's room. My sister told us she would say good night to my mother and find out what the noise was so I could get ready for bed. I didn't get ready for bed but let her check on my mother. I knew she was up or there wouldn't have been any noise. I then heard my sister through the monitor telling my mother to get her gown back on her. It was late and bedtime. My mother told her to mind her own business and get out of her bedroom. She told her she was the boss of the house and she would get dressed if she wanted. I sat down and made myself comfortable. I wanted to see how long it took for my sister to convince my mother that it was dark outside the house and bedtime. Alzheimer's patients don't go by time.

After listening to them for 20 minutes, with my sister thoroughly upset and mad herself, I went into the room. My mother looked up and said, "There you are. Tell her to leave." So I told my sister to go home and thanked her for the two and half hours of help. My sister said that maybe she would go to sleep for me. I was irritated. I told my sister that she will be up for another couple of hours because she was dressed at 10:30 p.m. Before we left for the party, I told my sister to check on my mother every 20 minutes, after she thought she was asleep and not to leave her alone in her room until she was asleep. But after my mother got into bed, she never went back into her room to check on her. My mother had been busy getting dressed, and no one knew it.

I didn't stress it enough, I guess. My sister still thought the television monitor was a little overboard, but hearing that first sound in her room or kitchen I would have been there instantly and hopefully would have prevented what occurred.

The next morning my mother got up early but was tired. She sat in her chair petting the dog. I was in the kitchen when she yelled, "Is my dog in there?" I told her the dog was on the floor next to her chair. My mother looked down and was relieved the dog wasn't lost. She had a cold stare and must have been in another world or time. Even though it was funny, I didn't laugh. It would have embarrassed her. I thought it was funny she asked about the dog even though she was petting it.

She was tired most of the day with very little talking or arguing. I was grateful because after the ordeal the night before, I couldn't handle a lot of activity. We were up late because my mother "had someplace to go" that night, after my sister had left. She just couldn't get the plans straight. All night she repeated that she had to go somewhere.

Chapter 3
Entering Her World

Just as time means nothing to babies, it means nothing to Alzheimer's patients. There were days when my mother would be in her night gown all day thinking it was evening and change right before bed to go shopping. I learned, after caring for her, that there was no rhyme or reason to their behavior. It was what it was. I had to accept that. I had to enter her world and leave mine behind. I got so good at being in her world that my husband had to ask where I was sometimes.

"Therapeutic Fibbing"

As I climbed into bed, my husband asked me something. I told him that my brain is dead and I didn't know what he was saying. I told him my body felt like it didn't belong to me; that I needed to get some sleep. I had to prepare for when my mother was awake. I will have to begin "therapeutic fibbing" again tomorrow.

"Therapeutic fibbing" is the term used by some Alzheimer's doctors. It became one of the hardest parts of caring for my mother. I have become better at it as I cared for my mother longer. I could tell when the anger rose, along with confusion and fear. It became necessary to enter her world and agree with her as long as there was no risk involved.

For instance, if she believed someone was alive, they were alive. If she had no children, she didn't have any children. After the first year, I found no good reason to make her mad by insisting on the truth, because the "truth" didn't exist in her world. Even though some doctors tell a caregiver to stand firm, I challenged them to stay in the same house with an Alzheimer's patient for two years and see how long they insisted on reality. I didn't think reality was as important to me any longer. I wanted to keep her safe and happy. That was all that mattered to me when I cared for her. The diseased person won't ever leave the home or care facility. Patients ought to be happy, and it's easier on the caregiver as long as there's no risk or harm to the patient. I might be wrong, but this seemed to be the best way for us to live with this disease.

Where Are the Cookies?

After reminding her again today where the bathroom was, my mother came out and said, "I don't know how I got here. Will you take me home?"

I always tried my best to remain calm and patient and explain she was home. I would try to change the subject. I poured a cup of coffee to try to get her to sit. I never knew if she wanted it with cream, black or none at all. Some times she couldn't remember ever drinking coffee. Today, she said to me, "Why did you pour me a cup of coffee? You know I've never been a coffee drinker." I answered, "Mom, try it with me. I promise you'll like it." She drank the coffee and said, "If you put a little more milk in it, I would like it better."

She smiled and I was glad to see her happy because it wouldn't last long. I always took every minute I could get.

My mother had to remind me, "You know when someone is offered coffee, she also is offered a cookie."

I said, "Of course Mom. How inconsiderate of me." I never bothered to tell her that she had just had a bowl of cereal for breakfast five minutes before then. This is how we began our day. The morning ritual lasted longer on some days than others. I used a lot of my energy trying to outwit my mother to keep her from getting upset.

My mother lived with us one and a half years before she went to be with my father; "Her Man" as she called him. She couldn't remember his name toward the end or what a husband was. In her mind, however, my husband and I lived with my mother, not the other way around. We also had to enter her world because it was easier for us to deal with her that way.

The White Plate

Over the last few weeks, I noticed my mother was slower when she came into the kitchen in the evenings. She wanted to put the forks on the table. I had the plates already on the table. She asked where I kept the forks. I showed her, as I did every night, and handed them to her. She placed them by the plates and asked to cook. I talked to her about the meatloaf that was in the oven.

After a few minutes, my husband entered, and my mother hugged him. She had already hugged him about 10 times since we got home from work because my mother thought my husband was just getting home even though he had been in the yard, or in the bathroom each time.

Of course, this exchange saddened me. My mother didn't offer to hug me at all. She didn't know me. I had to be strong and not let her know I was sad. It was hard to deal with her not recognizing me as her daughter. At first, my husband would say, "Ruby, do you know who is standing over there? It's Linda." But my mother always answered, "No I don't. I haven't seen her in years." She never made the connection that we were even married. I wondered who she thought Rod was. He might have been one of her sons. She never said, but she did know him and liked him.

My sadness disappeared this evening at dinner, though. My mother picked up her fork and tried to stab the grapes that were painted on the plates. My husband and I looked at each other. We smiled, but soon, it hit us that she thought the grapes were real. I passed potatoes to her to distract her because she was getting annoyed at not being able to pick up a grape. She told me I could help her with the dishes since she cooked the meal.

The next day, I decided to buy a white plate for my mother to use. The new plate also was lighter in weight, which helped when she wanted to wash it in the sink after meals. We had noticed earlier that she was having trouble carrying the other plate to the sink. When we had finished our meals, we looked at each other smiling and asked her if she was going to finish the grapes. Her answer was, "You stinker." She smiled because the plate was empty and she could see the grapes were painted on the plate. Still, to this day, every once-in-a-while, my husband asks me if I'm going to eat my grapes. We always laugh.

The Last Shower

Today had been a normal day, so far. The pacing began at 4 p.m., as usual, but as I prepared dinner, this evening was a little different because Mom seemed less active. She wasn't walking or talking much. She stood in the kitchen just long enough at times for me to start something and finish it. Sometimes, just getting the lettuce washed took an hour. I thought she was tired this evening.

At dinner, she didn't eat much. I didn't get too excited about it. My husband told me she would eat when she was hungry. I left the kitchen to take her back to her room. She looked like she was falling asleep. I asked her, "Do you want to take a warm shower, Mom?" I didn't say anything about going to sleep because I didn't want her to worry. My mother said she wanted the shower.

I didn't realize that this would be her last shower alone. I helped her get undressed, but I didn't help with the underwear. She still knew enough to be embarrassed by her body. I turned on the water leaving the shower door open as usual. I told her I would be outside the door if she needed help. I stepped outside the door, sat on the floor and fell asleep.

When I realized I had fallen asleep from my fatigue, I asked Mom if she was ready to leave the shower. A soft yes came through the door. I will never forget the sound of her voice at this point. I jumped off the floor and ran in to see her standing in the shower shaking with the washcloth in her hand still dry. She said, "I don't know how I got in here and I don't know what to do!" She was so cold and nervous as I helped her out of the shower as fast as possible.

I called to my husband for help and threw towels around her. My husband helped me get her to her bedroom. My husband knew "the yell", as he called it, and threw everything aside to be at my side instantly.

I put my mother in her robe and rubbed her arms and legs with lotion. She soon forgot the matter but kept repeating, "I don't know how I got in here." I rubbed lotion on her back because she said it hurt. I started crying because I knew this would have to be her last shower alone. After that night, I had to stay in the bathroom by the shower door, and eventually washed her.

I was upset that my mother was cold and confused, but I think I was more upset that another task had been taken from her memory. A simple thing like a shower had to be explained to her. I had to show her again how to use the washcloth. I had to ensure the water was warm and not scalding when she showered.

After my mother was safely in bed, I sank in a small sofa in her room. I fell asleep again. I heard something and woke. My mother looked down at me. She said, "Are you going to spend the night with me?" I told her, "Yes, I believe I will."

"Then, I will give you a blanket," she said as my mother grabbed a blanket from the end of her bed and spread it over me.

"It's too late for you to drive home anyway." She sat in her rocker and smiled at me. She said, "Go to sleep. I love you."

I closed my eyes again but not to sleep. I wanted to think and cherish another great moment where I got my mother back for a few minutes, doing what she did best, caring for others. This was how I remembered her before the Alzheimer's took her memory.

As I lay there, I thought about it and took great pleasure of my mother comforting me like a child. I wondered if God was speaking to me. If He was, He said, "You couldn't prevent her from forgetting what to do in a shower."

These were the moments that brought me joy. I came to appreciate the little times she remembered me. They made up for staying up to 2:35 a.m. and for dealing with my mother's crazy moments.

The Purple Night Gown

My mother wasn't awake yet that morning, even though it was about the time she usually got out of bed. I laid her clothes on the chair in her room. I was trying not to wake her. The aid came at 8:00, as usual, so I could go to the office for four hours. I told her I laid out my mother's clothes and filled a bowl with cereal on the counter.

After the four hours, the aid was waiting for me at the back door. She wanted to talk to me privately. We were interrupted when my mother said, "Boy am I glad to see you." She breathed a heavy sigh and put her whole body into it. So I knew they must have had a difficult morning.

That day was the first of many days that my mother didn't get dressed. She had on her gown and her purse over her shoulder. After I talked to my mother for a few minutes, she went to sit in her gold rocking chair. I gave her a glass of tea, and she was relieved and more settled than when I got home. Although she didn't know me as her daughter, she somehow knew me as the one who lived in the house. I also hoped that she knew me as the one who protected her.

The aid told me that she went into my mother's room that morning and tried to help her get dressed into the clothes I had laid out. My mother said, "This is my house. I'll get my clothes on when I want. You can just leave." The aid had laughed to herself, went into the kitchen, cut my mother a piece of cake, poured coffee and took it into her bedroom. My mother had forgotten what happened and ate her cake. When she was ready to leave her bedroom, the aid asked her if she wanted to get dressed. My mother answered that she was dressed so that was the end of that.

For the rest of the day, my mother wore her gown. My husband came home and asked why she was ready for bed already. She had forgotten and looked at her robe with an expression of confusion. I didn't know how my mother was going to react. I reacted quickly and told her it was getting late. My mother didn't recognize time any more, but she always knew when it was meal time. I made sure dinner was at 5:30 every day because she had to take food with her heart medicine. I would give her small amounts of food on her plate. If her plate was full, she wouldn't accept it at all pushing it away, knowing she couldn't finish it.

When I brought the food, she had been petting her dog beside the rocker. Before eating, she wanted to wash her hands. Knowing that she had a difficult day and that I didn't want her to leave her chair, I went to the sink and got a wash cloth so she could wash her hands, after petting the dog. She ate, but not much. Then she started pacing and wondering if the doors were locked. By nine, she was so very tired. I helped wash her face, and she fell into bed. I rubbed her legs with lotion because they were swollen. She continued to worry about the doors even after she fell asleep. At times, she jumped up and asked about the doors. She wanted to check on them herself.

I told my husband that she won't stop thinking about the doors. I was mad that her memory had failed her and could only give her fear and confusion. I cried for a long time. But my husband reassured me that she was being cared for better at my house than in a facility. He told me to get rest because I would need it the next day. Before I slept, I checked on her. She was asleep. I was also able to sleep, but I never knew how long because she often woke in the middle of the night.

I learned that night doesn't mean sleep to an Alzheimer's patient. Night only brings a fear like nothing else. It's as if she was dropped onto this planet. She wasn't familiar with it and had no

59

knowledge or concept of anything. Nothing has meaning. Alzheimer's patients are hunting for a place to rest, but they can't find it.

I found it strange that my mother was worried about having a place to sleep, but she never thought she was tired enough to go to bed. Many nights after the "sun-downer" pacing stopped, or her swollen legs and feet brought it to an end, we couldn't get her to sit down. My mother couldn't walk many times. She would hold on to the door, chair, or stair rail. She leaned against the wall in the hallway as she paced, because of swollen feet.

My husband said the pacing was her job. He said this was what Alzheimer's patients do, and my mother did her job well. She would pace nonstop until her feet couldn't take another step. On many nights, neither could mine. She was looking for a bed and something familiar. She looked every night, but never found it, something that was never lost in the first place. That day was different, because she wore her gown all day, but never knew it.

Television

One September, I remember the temperature was around 103 degrees outside the house, but my mother was cold. She sat in her gold chair in the family room, with blankets wrapped around her shoulders and across her legs. She was fully dressed with pants, tube socks, blue tennis shoes, and a sweatshirt that all matched, but one would never know under those two blankets.

She spoke little as she sat looking out the window in her cold stare. At times, I stood in front of her to see if she was okay, in a coma state at times. Not eating much or drinking, so only a few times did she request assistance in helping her to stand up so she could go to the bathroom. I had to lean over so she could grab my neck for her to stand, each day getting harder for me because I could feel more of her weight as I helped raise her.

Bedtime came early for a change. My mother did little pacing. She was tired. She asked me to show her the gown. It was an unusual day. That night I sat with her in her room watching television and she was still quiet for some time. Then, looking up from her rocking chair, she stopped rocking and said, "Is there anyone still alive that I still know?" and "What will happen to me?"

As we talked, I answered her questions with, "yes there are many people still alive, but you don't like driving much, and you live with me because I insisted on it." I knew I had to get her off that subject or she would be upset right there at bedtime. After telling her some friends would be by tomorrow to visit, she willingly went to bed. I used another "therapeutic fib". I straightened her pillows and hugged her a dozen times; otherwise she'd be up in five minutes when the lights were turned off. Again, I said, "You live here with Rod and Linda. We love you so very much, Mom." I repeated "Rod and Linda" at least four times then she sat straight up in bed looked at me in the eyes which she had not done all day and said with a big smile, "You're Linda." I told her I was. It felt good to say "Mom" so I said it again smiling as big as she had. She said, "Well, I can go to bed now and sleep." But she got out of bed, took my graduation picture off her dresser and put it in the center of her bookshelf where she could see it. She said the picture was her when she was young. Then she said, "I must be really old because right now you look old." I didn't know whether to laugh or cry.

As I was leaving her room, she asked me where all those people were who were in the room talking. It took me a few minutes to figure out that she was talking about the television. I told her they went home to bed, and she liked that explanation.

I kissed her good night again, and she said, "What would I do without you?" I told her we would always be here for her. My mother smiled and closed her eyes, nodding her head. I sat by her for a while to make sure she was asleep this time. I also went over her words again and again in my mind. She had spoken my name. My mother remembered me as her daughter and she felt safe here. My job for the day was done. I went to bed to sleep. Having her feel safe gave me a good, warm feeling inside.

My husband and I laughed about me being old, and after looking back at my mother's younger pictures, I could see where she thought my graduation picture was her, but why she jumped up to get it was a puzzle.

It was a few weeks later as we watched television on our big screen and my mother started asking how the people got in there. At first, it amused us, but then if we noticed she was confused and became nervous, so then we would turn off the television. We would give her ice cream to distract her from the television. Ice cream was her new favorite food.

We had to become especially aware of her state of mind from then on. After the television was off, many times for up to an hour, she would still think there was someone in the house. She remembered the talking but had forgotten it was from the television set. Again, my husband was so tuned into my mother and caring for her that he gave up the sport and history channel for her, many days.

The television seldom got turned on in her bedroom after that. If I did watch the news in her room, I always made sure we had at least one to two hours before she went to bed.

My mother started spending more time going through her wallet and purse and jewelry box after the television thing. She would spend up to three hours sitting on the edge of bed or in her rocker going through her purse without moving. She never missed the television. I guess it was me who missed it the most. She couldn't miss anything she couldn't remember. She also spent a lot of time going through pictures. But as I looked at her eyes, I often wondered if she saw or knew who was in the picture; or she would hold the picture and look over it and over it without emotion. She clearly didn't know those people.

She became more withdrawn and quiet without talking. It was hard for me to deal with the silence, so I started taking that time in the evening to clean her room. It gave me something to do, as I sat with her before bed.

One evening as I had dusted her bookshelf, she quickly got up to rearrange it, of course. As she moved all the pictures around she said, "I don't know who all these people are but they keep sending me pictures so I have to put them up in case they come to visit me.

All she wanted was a face of someone she knew. She wanted people in her life, but they were taken from her. Such loneliness my mother felt, and I, to this day, cannot feel as she did. It's impossible for me to do so as I can not block my memory, believe me, I've tried to put myself in her shoes. So all those pictures of family members she was rearranging by herself was really no different than those people on the television set. She knew none of them.

Hair Washing

I was paying bills at the kitchen table. I saw my mother standing beside me with a blank look on her face. She asked if she could wash her hair because it hadn't been washed in a week. I told her of course, and I got her a towel. I knew she had washed it the day before. My husband had put a laundry tub in the laundry room because my mother would put her head under the kitchen faucet at all and odd times to wash her hair. We figured out the hair-washing thing would become her out, making her feel good.

Quickly, grabbing her arm as she went to the kitchen sink, I took my mother to the laundry tub where we had a generous supply of shampoo, conditioner and lots of towels. We would wash her hair once-a-day or up to four times a day. My daughter, many times, had to finish washing my mother's hair when she came to visit so I could go back to paying bills, laundry or other things like putting my clothes back in my closet that she got out that day or cleaning up the dog mess. She never cared who washed her hair.

I noticed the before and after-effects of hair-washing. These little details weren't real to us, but they were real to her. She would be nervous and sad. She would run her fingers through her hair, repeating over and over, "My hair hasn't been washed for weeks. Is there any place in this house I can wash my hair?" She acted like she wanted to reach for something that would make her all better and solve all of her problems.

After her hair was washed, blown dry and styled, her whole mood would change. She would say thank you many, many times and mumble over and over, "How good her head felt because it had been a week since her hair had been washed." She would tell me that there hadn't been any place to wash her hair. She made these comments even when we washed her hair two hours before this. We spent a lot of time at the laundry tub.

I realized that with her hair, as with other issues, the best answer was always yes. She loved the feeling of clean hair. I admit that when she first came with us, I had hoped she would stop wanting her hair washed. Instead of stopping, the requests became more frequent. I reminded myself time and again that we had to live in her world.

Another morning, my mother asked about washing her hair. I wanted her to eat her breakfast first, but she insisted she ate hours ago. I poured her some coffee and gave her a piece of toast. I said, "If you ate hours ago, you must be a little hungry. Have a piece of toast." Before she finished her toast, I was just as anxious to get her hair washed as she was because she repeated over and over, "my hair hasn't been washed in weeks."

We learned, after two years, that this activity would be a time of enjoyment for my mother. It would be an activity where there was no confusion, confrontation or anger. Hair-washing became sacred. When I would drive up to my parents' house, before they moved close to us, my father would always ask if I would wash my mother's hair. Before I cleaned or cooked, that would be the first thing I'd do. He said she complained constantly about her hair and even he, at times, helped wash her hair.

My Dog Is Starving

My mother and my husband were sitting at the table one evening. I had cleared it and was doing the dishes. She asked if we were going to eat tonight. My husband tried to explain that we had already eaten. He told her we had some leftovers if she was hungry. He didn't tell her we ate 10 minutes ago. She had enjoyed that meal. She told me that the green beans were good. But now the meal was forgotten.

She asked if we had anything sweet. I pointed to the cookie jar and told her it had her favorite peanut butter cookies. She took one to hide in her pocket and one to eat while standing in the kitchen. She'd forget about the other cookie. I knew I would find it the next day in the bathroom or somewhere else.

Then, she asked if we had food for the dog. This was the 20th time in the last hour she had asked about food for the dog. I knew

65

her dog wasn't hungry, but my husband put food in the dog's bowl. My mother insisted that my husband take it to the dog. My mother's dog looked away. My mother said the dog likes his food with gravy on it and that the dog was starving. At this point, I knew my husband wasn't getting anywhere close to satisfying my mother about feeding her dog who wasn't hungry. So I put down the dishes or dish towel and took my mother away from her dog. My husband helped by taking the dog outside the house, but it took 35 minutes of my mother saying her dog was starving before she moved to another subject.

My younger granddaughter was so good with my mother. She had come over one morning to take the dog for a walk, but as she stood by the front door with a cookie in her hand, my mother walked right over to her and took the cookie. She told her to go home, and my granddaughter stood there smiling and agreed, even though her feelings were hurt, and she had tears in her eyes. She would tell my mother that she wanted to take her dog for a walk. My mother would look at her dog and tell my granddaughter to be sure to bring the dog back.

Even though my mother didn't remember the people in her life, she remembered her dog. She recognized her dog's tags that jingled when the dog moved. The sound drove me nuts but somehow gave my mother a feeling of security, so I dealt with it.

My mother stood looking out the window and said she needed to stay there so she could see her dog. When she couldn't see my granddaughter any more, my mother thought my granddaughter stole the dog. When my granddaughter came back with the dog, my mother greeted her at the door and asked how she would feel if someone took her dog without her knowing it, very rudely. My granddaughter was puzzled and told her she wouldn't like it. She said she would tell her the next time she took the dog for a walk. My mother thanked her and asked if the dog went with her willingly. She told my granddaughter to ask, next time, to take the dog.

It was amazing that at age 14 my granddaughter knew how to deal with someone who had no memory. I could always count on her to help with the dog, for the next two years. However, my granddaughter went longer between visits.

At the end of the day, my mother asked me again about scraps for the dog. I had already fed the dog. I knew this night would be a difficult one, because for the seventh time, my mother was in the kitchen setting all the food out on the floor. I called my husband and asked him to take the dog outside the house and distract my mother. I was tired. I finally had laid on my sofa in my family room so I could see her pacing back and forth. One time, she asked me if all I did is lie on the sofa and watch television. My body ached, and my eyelids were half closed. I said nothing, because at that moment, words would have been spoken that I would have regretted the next day.

She kept asking me about feeding her dog. I wanted the day to end. I told her a story. They were more "therapeutic fibs". I told her the dog was in her room and asked her if she wanted to get on her pajamas and call it a day. She told me that because I spent all day on the couch I should already be wearing my pajamas. I didn't get angry. I decided I needed to get her in her room, keep the dog away from her, get her nightgown on her, and give her a sleeping pill. All day she had been feeding the dog.

Of course, my husband laughed at my mother's witty saying. I got mad at him, but that evening after she went to bed, I could laugh with him.

Stolen Purse

I walked my mother back to her bedroom, hoping to help her get dressed. She did. Before I could get her back to the living room she said, "I can't find my purse." I thought, "Oh no." I was worried because I knew the aid was coming soon and I wasn't ready for work yet. In my mother's world, her purse was a big deal.

We began to search. We looked everywhere but couldn't find it. Usually, at night, after she had gone to sleep, I would put her purse in her top drawer. I was sure I had that night too. My mother must have gotten up during the night and gotten it out of the drawer before coming into the kitchen. It was gone. We tore the bedroom apart.

The aid came into the room and said softly, "I'm here." My mother heard her and asked, "Who was that?" She said to keep her from her room. "She probably took my purse." The aid had heard this many times and knew not to say anything. She wanted to solve this purse problem more than I did. I'd be leaving for work and she would be the one listening to my mother say over and over about someone stealing her purse and money. My mother would go from room to room making sure the doors were all locked. The aid knew this could be a day, like others, when my mother would stand in the living room afraid and shaking. The whole time, she would think, "someone will break into my house," because of her purse being missing.

I knew we had to find the purse, and fast. We looked under the bed, between the mattress, in all the drawers, in her trunk, in the sofa, and in her closet. It wasn't in any of these places. I decided that she must have been up in the middle of the night and in the small bedroom next to hers. I asked the aid to go into the small bedroom and look. It was in the closet, under some blankets. I was amazed that she was up in the middle of the night and made it back to her room.

I took the purse from the aid without her seeing it and told my mother I found it in the bathroom. She assumed someone wanted to take it, and dropped it as they were leaving, after breaking into the house. I told her we didn't put it in her room when we came home last night but left it in the bathroom. This got her mind off the "stranger" in the house. The aid was relieved and thanked me for staying until we found it. The aid was afraid my mother would lock her out of the house. I told the aid to keep my mother's mind off strangers in the house. I told her I had washed her hair already this morning and to put the house key on her arm in case my mother locked her out the house.

When she was afraid of strangers in the house, a feeling that could come at any time for no reason, my mother always walked up and down the hall, closing and locking all bedroom and bathroom doors. She also always locked the outside doors and would go back to make sure she hadn't forgotten one. Of course, this meant we had to keep up with her.

Flower Pots

The aid met me at the back door when I came home from work and told me my mother was upset and angry all day. She was being harmful and also pushing. The aid didn't get too close to my mother and allowed my mother to be the boss. My mother told her to get out of her house, but the aid didn't, of course. Instead, she walked to the pantry or the laundry room and closed the door, but she left it open a crack so she could see her. My husband came home early and tried to calm her. It didn't work. He went to the bedroom to read, hoping the aid could handle it earlier in the day.

After the aid left, my mother asked me if my husband had died, several times. I took my mother back to her bedroom to lie down. She was drained from a difficult day. She couldn't remember anything that happened. I checked on her to make sure she was asleep. Several hours later, I asked my husband to read in the living room while I went grocery shopping for an hour. This way, he would be able to see my mother if she got up.

When I came home, I had bags of groceries in my arms and noticed something red out of the corner of my eye. I put down the groceries and stepped into the living room. Potted red geraniums were sitting all over my living room, on the floor, on the coffee table and on the end tables. I yelled at my husband, wondering what happened in the 60 minutes, or fewer, I had been gone. My husband jumped off the couch and looked around. He said he must have fallen asleep. I yelled again, saying, "You can't help me with my mother for an hour without sleeping?" She had brought in all these potted plants and opened and shut the door several times. I asked my husband if he could hear. Then, sarcastically, I said, "obviously not."

My mother heard us arguing and came to us to say if we wanted to argue, we should go home. She looked at the plants and said if we wanted to bring all the flowers in the house, we should have them in one place. They would be easier to water, she thought. I was angry about mulch being on my floor. I said nothing to my mother. My husband told me he would get the groceries while I cleaned up the mess.

We carried the plants back outside the house. My mother wanted to keep some in the house because it was going to freeze tonight. It was May in Arizona. I knew there was no chance of frost. This was one time I forcefully did what had to be done, even though I knew she would be mad. The mulch all over the living room carpet was more than I could handle.

By dinner, my mother had forgotten all about the flower episode. My husband apologized several times for falling asleep. I got the carpet shampooed to get out the wet mulch and potting soil out of my rug.

Paper Towels

When I came home from work, I asked my mother if she had missed me. I asked her that every day. Her reply was, "Fine thing you did leaving me hear all alone all day. Where have you been?"

The nurse told me it had been a good day, which I didn't hear that often. I was pleased. The rest of the day was good also. My mother got dressed several times by herself and changed shoes every 15 minutes. She was busy. I noticed a half sheet of paper towel rolled up in her hand. It was dirty. It could have been one she hid in her trunk or shoe boxes. I asked her to come to the kitchen sink that I wanted to show her something. I wanted her to wash her hands with soap. She got upset when I tried to remove the paper towel from her hand. She was worried about the paper towel, like it had feelings. I finally got her hands washed, and gave her a new paper towel. She wanted the old one. I gave her back the old one, but I put a clean one in my pocket so I could exchange it for the dirty one when the time was right. Something like a paper towel meant so much to my mother. I couldn't understand that.

Horses

One evening, after my mother was in her bed, I sat on her bed. We heard the neighbor taking his trash can to the road for pickup the next day. His driveway was close to my mother's bedroom window so she could hear the wheels of the trash can as he rolled

71

it over the gravel driveway. It was a familiar sound, but I had heard it many times before this. I didn't pay much attention to it. On this night, as my mother heard the noise, she said, "Boy. The neighbors are sure hooking their team of horses up late to go into town. I hope everything is all right." I thought a few minutes and realized she was thinking she was back on the farm with horses. After we had talked a few more minutes, she asked me if I had fed the horses yet. I asked her what horses. She told me the horses that were in the back of the barn. I told her I fed them and all the other livestock. I didn't know if my mother would think there were other animals.

Several weeks later, as she lay in bed, almost asleep, the neighbor pushed his trash can across the gravel drive to the street again. She jumped in bed and asked if I fed the horses. I told her I did, but this started a regular routine with my mother whenever she heard the trash can on the gravel.

One evening my mother was really nervous. She was worried about everything, and she heard the trash can again. She asked if I had fed the horses. I was tired and was afraid she was going to make me check on the horses as she had done in the past. I told her a "therapeutic fib". I said, "We sold the horses and bought a car." I laughed, thinking I sounded ridiculous and that she wouldn't believe me. I wasn't sure she even knew what a car was. Her answer made me laugh harder. She said, "Good I was tired of feeding the horses every day." She went right to sleep.

The Wedding Plans

Just yesterday, I had to help my mother with moving around the house. She used her cane somewhat. She was getting weak. I had to help her eat and get into bed. Now, today, she woke, angry and full of energy. She started pacing early in the afternoon.

She didn't sit down for hours at a time. That worried us. We were afraid she would fall. Her anger had changed into fear, asking us where she was going to sleep. She said, "You moved me here without my permission. Now where will I sleep?"

I showed her to the bedroom, but she would forget instantly and walk right back out the room. She repeated this ritual over and over. We decided to give my mother a sleeping pill. Her doctor said my mother could have a pill every other night and probably should. Many nights, we chose not to give it to her. My mother never took medicine and I wanted to keep it that way, as much as possible.

Two hours after the sleeping pill was given, she was still pacing the floor. Her body didn't slow down like it had other nights after taking the pill.

After wondering where she would sleep, my mother started wondering about getting ready for a wedding. She asked me to help her get ready for the wedding, that there was so much to do. My husband and I were stunned. We didn't know where my mother got this at 9:30 in the evening. He said, "You two girls go ahead and get ready for the wedding. Let me know when to be there. I'm going to bed now." He shut the bedroom door. I realized I was on my own this night. Of course, I smiled at what he said.

I tried to put everything back in her room as she pulled it out: flowers, purses, shoes and her address book. But I couldn't keep up with her energy. She opened her old antique trunk and started pulling out everything from it. She got out her suitcases. All of a sudden, she wanted to know where her kids were. I thought, "Oh great. Now I have to talk about my brothers and sisters. I wanted to wring their necks at that point for not being there to help me." My mother asked me again about her kids and told me to call them. I was glad we were off the wedding. I thought maybe she would slow down and I could sit and rest.

As we talked about the kids, I realized that, in my mother's mind, her children were young. She wanted me to get them. She said she could take care of her own children. I prayed that I wouldn't say "Mom" to her because she wouldn't understand since her children were babies. I wasn't even born yet, in her mind.

Not very often was I at a loss for words, but I was this night. I explained that her babies were spending the night at their grandparents' house. My mother continued over and over with this.

I let her talk. She changed the subject from one thing to another so fast. I didn't want to get her more upset, or angry than she already was. I was confused and very tired. I sat on the sofa, she told me to get up because there was stuff to do. She talked about Alfred. She knew he was her husband. I knew her mind was back many years. She had small babies and a wedding to plan. She was moving tonight. I wondered later what part of this long evening was real at one time and what part was fiction.

At 1:30 a.m. when I got her into bed that night for the last time, she told me she was glad I was there to help her. She said she had a lot to do to get ready for the wedding tomorrow. I said, "Yes, I have things to do, such as go to bed and get some sleep." She got angry at me and sat up in bed. I knew I had said the wrong thing. I then told her, "We need rest to get everything done for tomorrow." I sat with her a little longer and she went to sleep. Thirty minutes later, she was up again. Around four in the morning, my mother finally fell asleep. My husband asked me if I got the wedding all planned when I came to bed. He thought he was funny, but, at this time, I didn't.

The Keys

My mother got dressed that day at 5 p.m. when I was starting dinner. I wondered if she realized it was dinner and not breakfast. Food didn't make sense to her any more. After I got dinner started, I went into her bedroom to see if she was OK. She was dressed with her purse out and going through it. I went back to the family room and turned on the television. She came out of her room, walked around the sofa, where I sat trying to find the news, and went into the kitchen. I jumped up quickly and ran into the kitchen. She stood in the pantry. She went back to her bedroom. I went back to finding the news station, after I checked on dinner.

She came back into the room and asked if I could get her something to eat. She looked around the house looking for something familiar. She answered her own question, "No. You just go about your business and leave me like you always do and never talk to me." She was mad for about 10 minutes, saying there wasn't food in the house, and no one ever talks to her. As I tried to talk to her, I realized she never heard a word I said. She repeated herself over and over. I'm not sure she even knew what she was saying. I didn't get to hear the news again that night. My husband came home as all this was happening and said, "You don't need to hear any news. There's enough going on in this house."

My mother didn't eat much as she sat at the table with her purse around her shoulder. I found it strange that my mother's dog sat right next to her on the floor. Before, she was always worried about feeding the dog, but her memory had weakened to the point where she didn't think about feeding it or hiding food for the dog in her purse any more.

At bedtime, she was confused. My husband believed it was going to be a long night if I couldn't get her to settle down a bit.

It took me an hour to get her gown on her. It was sad because she only got dressed a few hours before I had to put her back into her gown. My mother started shaking. I hated it when this happened because she got so scared. She sat on her bed, but refused to get into it. She asked me where the girl was that was just here. I didn't know whether she talked about her school days or something else. I told my mother she went home. Then, my mother asked about the keys. I quickly told her I put them in her purse. My mother still carried her purse even though she had her gown on her. She looked through her purse but asked about Alfred. She said he was just there giving her keys. She asked where Mary was, who also was just here. I went along with whatever she said. She talked about seeing things that I couldn't see in the room. This was a new phenomenon to me.

When I asked her to lie down, she told me she wasn't tired. She told me to go to bed. Every time she asked me to go to bed, I wished I could. I didn't want to go to bed, however, because I knew there was a tomorrow. There would be two tired people who must deal with each other. My mother, on the other hand, didn't know there would be a tomorrow. She lived in the present and that was sometimes too hard to deal with.

Later in the night, her speech slurred. I thought it was because she was tired. She tried to get up but it was difficult for her to stand straight or walk. It took both my husband and me to keep her down. We didn't want her to fall and hurt herself that night.

We sat in her room. If she got up, we jumped to grab her or ask her what she needed. I said, "I'll get it for you." Most of the time, she would look at us with a blank look and say she didn't know why she got out of bed, that she couldn't remember. She would sit down on the side of the bed and then lie down. She never really slept. I stayed with her all night.

The Rest Stop

One morning, as my mother and I sat at the kitchen table, she asked me, "When are we leaving here?" I didn't want to upset her so early. I assumed she was talking about going home again. I answered, "Can we just sit here for a while and finish breakfast?" She said, "We only pulled over to rest for a while because Alfred was so tired from driving and now we've been sitting here at this roadside table for a long time."

I realized she wasn't even at the same table where I was sitting this morning. Alzheimer's patients don't always see what we see, even right in front of us. My mother was on a long road trip in Arkansas, somewhere sitting at a roadside rest stop table. I was in my kitchen eating breakfast in Arizona.

After we sat there for a while longer, talking about the trip, I told my mother I would go over to the car and make sure we had everything. She asked about Alfred again. I went outside for a few minutes and by the time, I got back in the house, she had moved from the table. It was all forgotten and now was lost again at another time, and in another place.

That is why I have said, so many times, that Alzheimer's patients can't be held responsible for their behavior. They are living in a past world, most of the time made up of childhood; past experiences of other people and that they aren't even themselves sometimes. There are things that happen to other people and because they remember it being stored somewhere in their brain they think it must be true. I am saying this from my own experience living with my mother.

So many times, my mother thought there were strangers in the house, especially in the bathroom or bedroom. Many times too, she said, she was talking to other people who weren't there. We couldn't see them but she did. Often, she talked of her conversations with people who have died.

In her last few months, she talked a lot to her deceased sister. She would tell me of their conversations and I would nod my head at first thinking, "OK." But after awhile, I got used to it. I never encouraged it, but, at the same time, I always let her finish her conversation, agreed and went on to the next topic. Sometimes, that was a conversation with another deceased person. She also said she talked to God or Jesus. My mother was a praying woman, so that didn't bother me as much. It became normal for her to talk to dead people or maybe, I should say, I accepted it so it became a little more normal for me to hear.

Sheets

This morning started out well. I got the sheets off my mother's bed while she was in the bathroom and her bedspread back on before she came back out. Sheets were a tricky thing around my house. If my mother saw me taking them off her bed, she would think I was stealing them. If I asked her to change them, she said, "No, leave my sheets alone. I only washed them yesterday, so they are clean." The sheets got washed every Monday and Thursday, and it was an all-day ordeal. It didn't help to have several sets because no one was fast enough to get the dirty ones off and clean ones back on the bed before she came back into the room.

When my niece came into the room, I told her half the task was done. The sheets were in the washer. My niece was pleased. Now, it would be her job to get them back on the bed peacefully. When I came home from work, I saw all my clothes on the kitchen table. I couldn't see anyone, but I heard music playing. I didn't see my niece, so I hurried to the back of the house to my mother's room.

My niece was putting the bedspread back on the bed and she was smiling because it was done. She said, "Grandma is resting in her chair listening to music she loves." I said, "Oh no, she's not. We have to find her." But I knew where she would be because all my clothes were on the table so she must be in my room, and she was. My mother could be as quiet as a church mouse. Today, she was. She had to have made at least three trips from my closet to the kitchen, because it took me three trips to return all my clothes back to my closet. I was happy they were still on the hangers.

My niece said, "Grandma, what are you doing? These are Aunt Linda's clothes. You went into her room and closet and got them out." My mother looked at my niece and said, "I haven't seen Linda for years, and I don't know who these clothes belong to, but they don't fit me so they are going outside. This is my house and I don't know who put them here, but I don't want them."

I stood there listening to them talk about me and my clothes thinking, "When do I get to say something?" But I knew it wouldn't do any good. I asked my niece to take my mother back to her room so she could go through her purse or count her shoes. I couldn't let her see me put the clothes back.

When they came back out, my mother heard the music and asked, "Can I sit down here and listen to this?" I said, "Oh yes. You can. I just might sit down and listen to it for a while myself." My niece stayed until I got my clothes hung in the closet. My mother had forgotten the clothes thing. Earlier that day, my niece said my mother was in my room going through my jewelry box, taking out all my necklaces and watches. She told her this was

Linda's room and my mother got angry with her, saying it was her room. It took a long time to get her out of my room.

Chapter 4
Overwhelming Tasks and Helplessness

Alzheimer's patients have trouble doing the most mundane tasks. These are the routine tasks we tend to take for granted. We just do them every day without thinking about them, such as brushing our teeth or pouring a bowl of cereal. At some point, the patients can no longer do these things. The caregivers have to be on alert for when that period of helplessness occurs and be able to adapt. In some cases, they have to adapt on a daily basis.

The Toothbrush

My mother asked me about her toothbrush. She wanted to know whether she had one. I showed her where it was and got her the toothpaste. She was confused, thinking the brush was mine. I learned from experience to set hers apart. I wrapped hers in a blue wash cloth. She somehow remembered her brush would be wrapped in a wash cloth. She got excited when she saw the wash cloth because she knew that was her brush. I also learned to use the same color toothbrush. In this case, I gave her a red one. I also used red Colgate toothpaste for her. I had several new red toothbrushes, in case she wouldn't believe the old one was hers.

It was hard getting used to her not knowing what items were and repeating activities, such as brushing teeth over and over. She would have to brush her teeth up to seven times a day because she couldn't remember having done it. Before, brushing her teeth brought her joy. It brought something familiar to her, in her mind. Her joy would only last for a few minutes, though.

After she was done, she wouldn't remember how to get back to the living room or her bedroom. I would wait and help her get back. When I couldn't wait for her, like when the door bell or phone rang, I would find my mother standing near the bathroom, or hallway, and shaking. She also wondered into all four bedrooms off the hall. I had a rule in my house that she was never to be left alone. I told the nurse, who came four days a week for four hours each, and the volunteers from our church who came to help, for about two hours a week, to stay with her always. If she didn't want them to stay then, they could hide from her sight but still be able to see her. I saw no reason to have my mother standing alone and scared.

Where Is the Trash Can?

My mother was in her bedroom going from picture to picture, mumbling. I went to ask my niece why the banana peels were in the back yard, for the last few days. My niece ran out the door and laughed that my mother had carried a banana all day, but she had never eaten it. We saw both banana peels and apple cores in the yard. My mother came shuffling out to the yard and told us we needed a trash can for the banana peels and apple cores. My niece and I looked at each other, grinned, and cleaned up the mess.

This ritual continued for two months. We found all left over food put behind the washer and dryer, in the washer, behind the sofa, but mostly out the back door. Eventually, she left it on the kitchen table as it got harder for her to get around the house. I never understood why she threw the garbage out the back door, but it could be because my mother used to burn her trash when she was young.

The funny part was that my mother scolded the people that were "creating the mess". She said, "Those awful grown people who leave a mess like this are wrong." I assumed she thought we did the mess because we were standing there. My mother looked at me and whispered that "she" was over here again. She pointed to my niece. At that, my niece knew she better leave before more things were said. My mother was bound to get angrier, or my niece was going to get more hurt. We needed to separate them. My niece left and my mother went back to her room.

When she got back to her room, she saw the pictures lying on her sofa. She said there must be a stranger in the house. I helped her put them back on her shelves. She blamed my niece for doing the mess in her bedroom. I noticed my mother was getting more and more upset, so I quickly put the pictures standing up right and not caring if they were in the right places. I knew she would move them later anyway. I had hoped that putting the pictures upright would end the confusion so we could move on to the next issue. My mother asked for a bathroom, and I knew that would take her mind off an intruder in her room. After taking her to the bathroom, I talked her into cookies and milk and side-tracked her mind even more. My niece had been the "intruder". She had forgotten who it was, only that someone must have been in her room.

Unfortunately, the distractions only lasted a little while. My mother asked my husband to take her home because someone here kept taking her things. I put on her music to calm her and did the laundry. I kept out of her way, but I had positioned myself where I could see her at all times.

Alzheimer's patients seem to worry about people taking their things quite a bit. I think the "things" represent a piece of themselves. This continued until late in the evening.

She stayed mad at someone but couldn't remember who. It was never good thing if she thought I was an intruder or person taking her things. I hoped her purse would have distracted her, as my husband asked her how much money she had. She would start to count it over and over.

Difficulty in Walking

It was a beautiful late afternoon, on a Saturday in September. It was the perfect weather for grilling. It also was an uneventful day, with mom sitting in her chair looking out the window most of the day. I had a good feeling about cooking outside. I knew she could see me from her chair without having to get up. That made me feel more at ease because I knew what could happen inside the house when I didn't keep an eye on her at all times.

Two of my teenage grandchildren rode their bikes to my house, after their ball game. I invited them to stay and eat. They said they would see how it went with their great-grandmother.

I asked one of them to go in the house to get the cheese for the hamburgers and look in on my mother. When he came back outside the house, he told me she was walking to her room. About 10 minutes later, I entered the house with the meat. I fixed my mother's hamburger first and put it on the table. I went to her bedroom to get her. She wasn't there. I screamed that my mother wasn't in her room. My daughter-in-law, who was just walking in the front door, ran out the door and scanned the street. My husband went out the back to look in the garage. My grandchildren and I started looking in the closets.

My husband found her in the guest room at the other end of the house, slumped over a sofa. Either she had fallen or was too tired to go on. We never found out the reason. She couldn't walk or move. My daughter-in-law got the wheel chair and we lifted her limp body into it. We pushed the wheel chair to the table to see if I could get her to drink something. It was so strange to see her eyes half closed and her head drooped. When I asked if she was hungry, she shook her head yes without speaking a word. Sitting right next to her, I gave her little bites of hamburger without bread. She ate a little and drank if I held the glass up to her just right. She spilled some on her lap, but I didn't care. I was glad to see she had an appetite.

When my grandson asked if anyone wanted the fries, my mother raised her hand as if she were in school. She ate a good portion of fries. Of course, the whole time, I was worried she was going to choke. According to the nurse, my mother could eat if she could swallow, but if swallowing was difficult, I had to stop feeding her. This would be our first time to hand-feed my mother.

We had pudding for dessert. My granddaughter asked if anyone wanted pudding. My mother raised her hand again without a word. We all laughed. She seemed to understand what we were saying. While my daughter-in-law fed my mother the pudding, I called hospice. The staff told me to get my mother into bed and stay with her. She should be different in a few hours, but if not, hospice would come and see her. I asked my mother if she wanted to go to bed and she nodded. I got her into bed, but it wasn't easy. My mother couldn't help me at all.

After washing her and putting her in her gown in her chair, my husband, my daughter-in-law, and I had to get her from the chair to the bed. This was the first time my mother wouldn't be able to stand. Many other times followed. As a result, getting my mother into bed became the most difficult thing, physically, that I would encounter.

As I reflect back on this, I wonder if my mother had a stroke or if the difficulty in standing was related to the Alzheimer's disease. I also found it odd that night to not see her pacing.

Loud Breath

It was the third day without sleep for me. My mother sat in her chair again. This was nice for me, but I knew things weren't right. She didn't want anything to eat all day or drink. She needed help going to the bathroom about every 45 minutes. If my mother didn't make it to the bathroom on time, it embarrassed her. She didn't want help either, but she had to have it. She couldn't bend over to change or even to find the clothes to wear. This had become a new issue for us.

This night, she told me people were in her room. She said she couldn't go to bed. Someone had gone into her room and stolen her purse and shoes. I finally got her ready for bed and into her room.

She had forgotten about the people and had asked me to find a knife she hid in the cushion of her chair. This surprised me. I never thought my mother thought about having a weapon for defense. I realized that what went through her mind wasn't normal. I shouldn't be surprised, because it really wasn't her. She insisted there was a knife in the room. She told me to find out who the people are, when they come back. She told me that I knew them. My mother turned the room upside down looking for a knife. I tried to change the subject, but I wasn't able to distract her. This lasted for more than an hour.

She then asked me why the room was messy. She wondered where the "baby" was. She said she was babysitting and had to find the baby. My mother got upset so I told her Rod took the baby for awhile. I said we would take the baby home soon. She seemed relaxed with those words. As we cleaned up the room, I knew I faced another long night. After a while, she sat talking about everything, jumping from one topic to another, sometimes in the same sentence.

The next day, the aid came as I was putting out my mother's breakfast bowl on the table. I asked her to take my mother a cup of coffee to her room before I left for work. She had come running back to the kitchen. She told me not to leave and to look at my mother. She was shaking really bad and said she was cold. She also was breathing really loud, almost puffing. I told the aid to sit with her and I called hospice. The nurse came immediately. We put blankets in the dryer to warm them and wrapped her in them. For the first time, my mother cried. She was scared, so I sat next to her, hugging her. The nurse took her blood pressure. It was low. I called work and told the office I would either be in late or not at all.

We continued covering her with blankets until noon. The nurse stayed with me. At noon, my mother stood and laughed like nothing happened because she didn't remember and asked why the woman was in her room. The nurse, at this time, decided to go.

Even though she was white as a sheet, and her lips were purple, she wouldn't sit. She got dressed slowly and even made her bed. She kept asking who all those people were. She also said she couldn't get around as much. My mother repeated this to herself, but she wasn't angry. The aid decided to leave too, when my mother started asking who the people were. I was scared. Her loud breathing still echoes in my head. She was unresponsive for three hours, except for the crying. Then she came back to us with no memory at all of the event.

Trouble Falling Asleep

My mother didn't know me that night. As I washed the dishes, she asked me who I was. She said she didn't know anyone in the house. She would stand close to me and not know where she was. I told her to stand by the sink next to me. She said the same thing over and over, because she was confused and afraid of her surroundings.

As I finished the dishes, I asked, "Mom do you know who I am?" That might not have been the best time to ask the question, but I thought it would bring her some piece of mind if she knew she was standing next to a relative. She told me no. I said that I'm Linda. She said she didn't know who I was, but my name was pretty.

That saddened me so much. All I wanted to do was to hug her and help her get memory back. I sympathized with how lost she must have felt. I hurried to finish the dishes because it was too late in the evening for her to get too frightened before bedtime. It also saddened me that even though she didn't know who I was, she approved of my name. Sadly, she never would remember that she was the one that gave me the name she liked.

I had to sit next to her that evening so she would keep her oxygen tube on her, for a few hours before bed. I don't know how much it helped. It was always such a fight to keep it on her. But we talked about good things a lot to calm her before bed. She kept talking about dogs and I thought she meant our dogs. But then my mother mentioned Bill. I wasn't sure what to say. I wasn't sure if she meant my brother who died at 35. I grabbed a picture off the shelf to show her. She said, "Yes. Bill. Where is he? He loves dogs doesn't he?" I told her he was at a friend's house.

Then my mother asked about Alfred. I wondered what to tell her then. He had died also. "Well," I said, "He and Rod went

WHY DO YOU CALL ME MOM?

fishing." Her reply was, "Why? I was just talking to him." She wasn't happy with my answer to this question. She insisted he was in the room and we were all talking. She repeated it several more times, so I said I would go look for him. I went down the hall, came back and told her they left to go fishing already. She had forgotten I told her the first time and was back on my deceased brother Bill.

This was the part of the disease I hated the most. I had to talk about people who were gone from this world, as if they were still here. I didn't really know what to do when my mother asked the questions. I knew I had to keep my mother calm and safe.

Because it was close to bedtime, I tried to change the subject and say something that made sense in her mind. Otherwise, I would have had to walk the floor with her all night. I told her again that my brother was staying at a friend's house. She asked when he would be back. I didn't know if she remembered him young or married, so I told her in about an hour. That satisfied her questions, but we went back to discussing Alfred. This back and forth continued for two hours. After that, she asked about feeding the dogs. I said they were fed and in the kitchen, or out back.

My husband came into the room to ask if he could turn off the hall light because it shined in his eyes in our bedroom. I told him I had to keep on the light, because my mother was afraid. I also asked him not to come into the bedroom, because he was supposed to be fishing with my father. If she doesn't remember my husband, she'll think he's a robber, breaking into the house. My husband looked at me like I was crazy, mumbled, "Sorry, I asked about the lights," and backed away into his bedroom.

My mother couldn't go to sleep that night. At 11p.m., as I laid on her sofa, I hoped she would fall asleep, but I was the one who fell asleep. She woke me by the sounds of her putting her shoes in her pillow case. She put them under the covers so no would take them from her that night. She said her plan was to leave in the morning. She said I could go with her. She was so confused and sad. I didn't want her to see me cry and bowed my head. I told her I would help her tomorrow after breakfast, that I loved her very much, and wouldn't let anyone hurt her. I could tell her body was so tired, but her mind was still going. I finally got her back into bed and covered. Her shoes were by her side. I kept telling her that I would be with her tomorrow. She finally fell asleep.

I told my husband how her body was too tired to move, but her mind was still active. I said I would have to go back to her room every few hours to make sure she wasn't scared in the night, even though I kept on the lights.

The next day was the same. She was mad at me for not taking her home. She stayed close to me because she said she didn't know anybody in this place. Everything got packed again, but she stayed on her bed. She was waiting for someone to pick her up. She said the person had called to tell her to be ready. I don't know if she remembered the phone or if she thought someone just hollered to her. I didn't dare ask.

When I told my husband, he said I was looking into it too much and not to worry about it. I told him I needed to know which it was so I could answer her questions and care for her better. He told me it would drive me crazy and tried to change the subject.

That second night she was up all night rearranging the pictures and talking to them. She told me to feed the dogs and horses because she didn't know where Alfred was. I decided to sleep in the back bedroom across from hers. That way, I was able to see if she got up and walked the hallway. Her dog also wouldn't let me sleep. He wore several tags that clicked and drove us all crazy, but we decided to keep the tags on the dog, because it was usually near my mother and the jingling sound gave us a warning if my mother was wandering the house. However, in the last few months of my mother's life, the dog seemed to need more sleep than she did.

The Conversations

There were only about four times that my mother got into our bed at night. The first shocked me because she woke me by pushing me over to the side of the bed. Instead of arguing, I let her lie there. She said, "I hope I didn't wake you, you fell asleep in my bed." She was so sweet about it. I couldn't make her go back to her room.

The other times she was so scared and shaking, that I didn't want to ask her if she was frightened in her room, or tell her that she was in my room. That would have embarrassed her and started an argument. Since it happened only a few times, we didn't make a big deal out of it. I assumed she thought she was in her own bed.

The things we noticed, in the later stages of Alzheimer's, were habits or practices of her earlier childhood. For instance, the last few months she would start looking for the dishpan at night and talk about watering the flowers at night. We thought this was strange, but found out later that when she was a child, she washed dishes in a dishpan and would throw the water on the flowers.

My mother forgot about most of her children except the oldest. For the last few months, she thought he was a baby. Before she died, she talked of him either being dead, or that he was in the room with her. She also talked about my late father being in the room with her. This became a daily topic about them.

She also talked about her sister being in the room. My aunt had died three years, before my mother, from Alzheimer's.

At first, these conversations she had concerned me, but the hospice nurse told me it was quite common. The nurse said, "Maybe, she's getting ready to leave this world. You should try to adjust to that idea also." Things started to change so fast toward the end. The last month, food meant nothing to her, except she liked pudding and ice cream. We would give her pudding and she would look at the spoon not knowing what to do with it. I didn't catch on right away. I would ask her if she was hungry. She would look at me strangely. When I took away the pudding, I could tell from her expression that she wanted it, but didn't know how to eat it. As I fed her the pudding, she would stick out her tongue when she didn't want any more. I was grateful because I knew when to stop feeding her and not force her to eat.

It also became hard for her to stand by herself. She walked with help up to the last week. She spent the last week in a wheelchair or in bed. That didn't sit well with her, though. She tried to get up so we had to sit right by the bed, full-time, because she forgot she didn't know how to walk.

The last few weeks were quiet. She didn't use words. The words she did use were confusing. I had trouble communicating with her. She shook her head a lot. I learned to read her thoughts through eye contact.

I will never forget the day she had to sit in a wheelchair, never to walk again. She had tried to stand beside the bed and fell back on the bed behind her. I got the wheelchair. She told me no, but I got her into it. I pushed her to the kitchen and made oatmeal cookies. She tried a hundred times to stand, and almost pushed out of the wheelchair. When I finally had the cookies made, I put one cookie and a glass of milk in front of her. She took one bite and frowned. I knew she was done eating. My daughter-in-law walked in the door and said, "Hi, Grandma." My mother looked up and motioned her to come close. She asked my daughter-in-law whether she could help her. Kathy told her to stay in the chair. My mother asked, "No. Can you help me go where I need to be?" We wondered where that would be, but we decided to take her back to her room.

After she fell asleep, I called the hospice nurse who came right over. My mother never got out of bed. The nurse said patients know when it's time to go. She didn't have to sit in the wheelchair that she hated anymore.

It was hard enough for her before, waking up in a house where she knew no one and everyone was a stranger. I knew she felt she was all alone in a strange place. As I saw her in bed, not being able to get up and run, as she had done before when she was afraid, I prayed that her mind was a little kinder to her. She wasn't able to walk or express her fears. Seeing her in bed, not communicating, knowing the fear that controls the mind was hard for me to take before she died. Today, there's not a doubt in my mind she is in heaven now, with a perfect memory and can name all of her children.

Chapter 5
A Feeling of Loneliness and Guilt

Keeping my mother calm, and in peace, always presented a balancing act. The job of taking care of an Alzheimer's patient is daunting, and at times, can be overwhelming. I had to find ways to let out my feelings without scaring my mother.

Moments to Myself

Some days, my mother would be angry. Some days, she would be sad and feel lost. I had to do my best to reassure her she was an important person in the house, with dignity, because I knew that was the way my mother would have treated me in the same circumstances.

Balancing these feelings against reality wasn't easy. I would go to the pantry and cry, when it became too much for me to handle. I would go to the bathroom just to sit down and rest. I always had to keep open the door enough to ensure my mother was in the living room.

At times, I wondered if my mother was the only person in the world experiencing this and I was the only person dealing with it. After I started to write out my thoughts in my journal and I talked to other people, I found it strange that there were so many people who had a relative with Alzheimer's, but they never told anyone. Some were close parents or grandparents. Those people didn't understand the disease, so we didn't talk about it at all. They said, "our grandparents have become mean, not wanting to have anything to do with our family. So we distance ourselves from them. There's no cure for Alzheimer's and we can't control them so we put them in a home, which is OK. They aren't to be left alone without someone monitoring their well-being and safety."

I couldn't think of anyone who said, "We tried to deal with Alzheimer's. We tried to understand how it changed our lives." I found most everyone telling me they blamed the person, not the disease, for the change in personality.

The Baby's Name

My daughter came over one day with my one-year-old granddaughter. My mother held the baby and played. She asked what the baby's name was. I said, "Lily." My mother didn't like that name. She said she was too sweet to have that name. My mother's aunt was named Lily. She was mean to everyone. No one liked my mother's aunt.

I realized I had to get my mother's mind off her aunt. This morning already was getting off to a bad start. My daughter never knew when she named their daughter Lily, which the name belonged to a dishonest aunt. My father told us the story shortly after my granddaughter was born. My mother got upset one day to the point of shaking.

My daughter took the baby from the room, and we decided to call her by her middle name, when the baby was around my mother.

While I made dinner, she asked me if my daughter was coming to the house today. My husband told her she came for a few minutes with the baby already this morning. I waved my hands at him not to call the baby Lily. He didn't, but he looked confused and told me to tell him later why I was waving my hands at him. He then was afraid to say our daughter's name too, not knowing what name I meant.

My mother said, "Well that stinker. She never came to see me." We had about 20 minutes of conversation, with my mother talking in clear words, not muffled together. It was pleasant. My mother loved being around babies and children under three years old. If they were older, she would always confront them about something, mostly food.

My mother laughed at dinner and ate well. My husband told me later that my mother was back with us for a short period. She even remembered that I was her daughter. Unfortunately, that was the last time.

We wondered if for a while, the baby brought back good memories, once we remembered not to call our granddaughter by her real name. I never met nor knew my mother's aunt.

The Sleeping Pill

The sleeping pill was difficult to get my mother to take because she told me she doesn't take any pills or vitamins so why would she take one after dark. I learned to use "therapeutic fibbing" and told her it was an aspirin for her legs that were hurting her. Of course, I wanted her to take the sleeping pill because she needed her rest. It was a difficult day.

My mother's doctor said my mother needed to take a sleeping pill every few nights, especially when she had been pacing or when the "sun-downer" incidents were bad. My mother had taken the sleeping pill hours ago, but it was after 11 p.m. and she still was in the kitchen putting food on the floor. It was chicken, hot dogs, and lunchmeat. I started to cry because I was tired. What she was doing didn't shock me at all. I had seen her do it other times. I was too tired to clean up the mess but knew I had to do it.

If I didn't clean up the meat, we would have stepped in it, or the dogs would have eaten it and gotten sick. Then I would have had to clean up the dogs' mess. I woke my husband and asked him to come into the kitchen. He put on some clothes and said, "Get your mother to bed. I'll clean up the mess."

She got mad and said, "Well, you didn't have to go tell him. You make it look like I've done something wrong." The last thing I wanted was for my mother to be upset, especially before going to bed. She would be shaking for hours. She was embarrassed and even though it was late, I felt sorry for her. It crushed my heart that she thought I was mad at her. I was wide awake now and realized I had to comfort my mother. She thought I wanted her to move out, so I laid across her bed telling her what a wonderful mother she was and how much she had helped me around the house and with the kids. My mother soon forgot why she was upset, sat up in bed, and asked about the scraps for the dog again.

I told her to go to sleep. To the dog, I said to come into the kitchen to get something to eat. I motioned to the dog, which was bloated already and ready to bust. My mother asked what she would do without me. As I walked out the room with the dog, it made me feel good. Of course, I didn't feed the dog any more food. After 10 minutes, I took the dog back to her room. My mother was almost asleep. I hoped this day would be over soon.

I don't understand why she got upset when she thought, that I thought, she had made the mess. She didn't want my husband to think she made the mess or he would force her to move out. When there was a conflict, my mother was afraid we would force her to leave. That was a horrible feeling to have. Even children don't believe they'll have to leave when they do something wrong. She felt lost most of the time.

My husband always made a point to let my mother know how much he loved her. He hugged her all the time and reassured her many times that her life was valuable, like saying, "Thank you Ruby for doing my laundry or helping with dinner tonight." He said these things even when she didn't help do those things. He wanted her to fell needed, as a person.

The Heart Attack

I had had a rough night. I couldn't get my mother to sleep before four in the morning. My husband let me sleep until six. He woke at five. I had two hours sleep. My mother slept until 10:30. Her nurse kept checking on her. When I got home from work at noon, my mother was ready to go again. She had her stuff packed in a pillow case.

I lied on the family room couch. She asked me if all I did was lay around the house. I answered, "Today, it is." I called my husband, asking him when he would be home because I was so exhausted. I couldn't talk. My mother wanted to talk, argue, and move. My husband said he would come home immediately. He wasn't feeling good himself. When he got home, we decided he should go to the hospital. I called someone to come and stay with my mother. My husband might be having a heart attack. He had heart problems. We sat in the emergency room all night. He was there all the next day. I didn't remember anything about the heart attack. I remembered about the incident, after I saw the bills in the mail.

After I got home, I went into my mother's room. She was sitting on the side of her bed and rubbing her face. I asked if her face hurt. She looked up and said she didn't know where she was.

I sat next to her thinking she must be so confused. I had been gone all day and my niece had stayed with her. I held her hand for an hour and hugged her. I told her she lived with me. She kept rubbing her face. As tired as I was, all I wanted to do was make her feel better about herself. I wanted her to stop being confused. After an hour, my mother wanted to know where her gown was. She tried to get up from the bed to look for her gown, but she wore her gown.

She looked down at herself when I told her she had her gown on and smiled. She said, "Silly me. No one took my gown after all." We laughed.

Mother would rub her face and neck a lot when she was worried about something. Maybe, she thought someone stole her gown, but she wouldn't ask my niece, or rather she didn't have a chance to ask her.

When we got home from the hospital, our bathroom door was open from our bedroom. I asked my niece about it. She tried to tell me a little that went on that day that my mother had run her husband off when he came over to eat dinner with them. He never got to eat because she thought he was stealing her food. He went to our bedroom to hide and watch television, thinking he would get food later. My mother found him, started yelling and we came in right after that.

My niece said it had been a normal day, with Grandma doing a lot of pacing, which made her tired early. Perhaps she was looking for me. All I know is she was so confused about where she was, what she was supposed to do next and couldn't find her gown that she was already wearing.

The "Neighbor"

On a Saturday, I heard my mother in the kitchen at 6 in the morning. I turned on the television camera in my bathroom, so I could see as I finished dressing. I wondered where she got her energy. I thought maybe we put too much emphasis on sleep. My body was tired this day. I willed my brain to work so I could protect and care for my mother. She only knew her mind had told her to get up so she was in the kitchen holding onto the counter. She wasn't able to move. Her body had betrayed her. Otherwise, she would know to sit down or not walk at all. I hurried to get the wheelchair.

As I grabbed the wheelchair, I prayed she didn't fall or try to walk. For the first time ever, my mother was barefoot. My mother never even went into the bathroom without her shoes. She went to the kitchen without shoes. I was saddened because she hadn't forgotten this minor point until now. Her feet must have been cold.

I knew something was wrong when I was helping her. She had lost another part of her memory. The other night, she wouldn't even walk from the bathroom to her bedroom without shoes on her feet, after getting ready for bed. I also noticed she didn't have her glasses either. I asked if she wanted her glasses. She looked at me strangely and asked me about glasses. I told her she wore them and realized she thought of a water glass when she asked me, how she would wear them.

My mother kept looking around the house. I wondered if she was looking for my father or someone she could trust. I asked her if she would like some coffee and told her to stay seated as she kept trying to stand. She just looked at me with sad eyes. I was sadder looking at her with bare feet and no glasses. I went back to her room to get her shoes and glasses. I wanted her to sit in her gold chair, not the wheel chair. She usually sat longer in her gold chair. She sat there most of the day wearing her gown, falling asleep on and off. When she was awake, she was angry and sad. She said she lived alone in the big house and no one ever came to see her, especially her children, if she had any that were alive.

When my husband came home that afternoon, I was putting hamburgers on the grill. Cooking outside was an outlet for me and I did it as much as I could. My husband yelled through the door to come into the house. Even though my mother could see me outside, at the grill through the French doors from her gold chair, she thought she was alone and was so frightened. My husband finished the hamburgers while I tried to comfort my mother. She shook for more than an hour repeating over and over the same thing   that she was alone.

She told my husband she had neighbors next door, but they never checked on her, as she lived alone. That made me feel awful. I was outside feeling good cooking, within a hollering distance, and she was inside frightened to death thinking she was alone. I was that "neighbor" who didn't care about her.

Chapter 6
Little Things Mean a Lot

When dealing with an Alzheimer's patient, short periods of lucid memories are treasured. These can get the caregiver through the tough times. In my case, my mother remembered her husband and she occasionally remembered her children's names. I also treasured my ability to care for her and not to have to send her to a facility.

She Remembered

My oldest son came over that morning because it was raining. He's a contractor. He can visit on rainy days, because they can't work outside. He told me that he hoped his grandmother would sleep through it. However, that didn't happen.

She came from her room and marched straight to my son. She held her head high and shoulders back. She was frowning with her mouth tightly closed. I feared what would happen next.

She looked right into his face bending down and then looked at my husband. She yelled, "How do you think it makes me feel to hear men talking in this kitchen and I come in here and Alfred is not here. My husband is dead and you two men just keep talking. I'm tired of it. Go away. I don't have a home."

They didn't say a word. They got up and walked out of the room. I went outside in the rain. I said to my son, "She's just sad over my dad passing away. She will forget after a few minutes. Please stay awhile longer and visit. I miss seeing my kids so much."

My mother watched him drive away, as I stood by the door. She asked me who was leaving. I said it was my son, Rich.

She looked at me with surprise and said, "Well, if that don't beat all. My own grandson came to my house and didn't even come in to see me." She remembered his name, but not his face.

I just looked at her, tears in my eyes, knowing how hurt my son must have felt. On the other hand, I couldn't be angry with my mother. I had to shake these hurt feelings so I could continue to protect her, even from herself.

That was one of the few times my mother said, Alfred. The rest of the time, she said, "a man" or "my man." Hearing my son and my husband talk loudly clicked something in her brain that brought back memories of her anger and sadness.

We went to her room. I helped her to get dressed and had only a few arguments. She tried to argue with me about clothes and shoes, but I answered only "OK" most of the time.

She said, "I'm so tired. Can I just sit here in my chair?"

After she was dressed and her bed was made, she sat in her chair. I brought her a cup of coffee in her room. I saw that my mother was breathing hard and that she was thinking too much. She had a cold stare. I realized that her memories were wearing her out physically. I talked to her. She only stared at me. I let her rest for awhile and was nervous about what to expect next. She was like that for several hours. She had nothing to say. I don't know what had happened, but she then started pacing. It continued the rest of the day.

Music as Therapy

This morning, my mother was dizzy and found it difficult to get to the table. I asked her if she wanted cereal and she looked at me puzzled, but she shook her head yes. She still was picking at her cereal and her coffee cup remained full when the aid arrived.

The aid asked me how my mother was. My mother gave her a blank look and wanted nothing to do with her. Knowing I had to go into the office for a few hours, I felt it would be best to get my mother back to her bedroom and helped her get dressed, without my mother seeing the aid again. My mother went down the hall angry, asking me who was this person and what was she doing there. Although the aid could hear the conversation, she was used to this treatment from my mother. She just smiled and cleared the breakfast food.

When I came home, the aid met me at the door. She told me my mother had a rough day and was angry and confused. She told the aid to go home every five minutes. My mother was in the hall. When she saw me, she asked, "Where is he?" I thought she meant the aid and asked who. She answered that he was in her room and said that he was coming for her and her things. My mother had thought my father was in the house.

I wondered how this conversation would end. We talked about my father being outside, working in the yard, and within a few minutes, her thoughts weren't on him as much as moving her things and who would help. I told her I would help, but it still didn't ease the situation. All she could think about was how hard moving was. She became more angry and confused. I try to get her from her room and away from her things, but it was hard. We went into the kitchen. She leaned on me and was shaking all over.

I sat her in a chair and got her something to drink. She wasn't interested. She wanted to go home.

I remembered that my mother enjoyed a country music CD that had no words to it. I quickly turned on the CD. After 10 minutes, she had relaxed into her gold chair as she listened to the soft music. I replayed it three times that afternoon. When music that had words was played, it didn't have the same effect on her as mellow music. Eventually, like with television, I played CD music less and less with the words, as it seemed to annoy my mother more than being a way to calm her. It was something she tried to understand, but it became an annoying noise to her.

The Smile

My mother had been thinking a lot about death lately. It might have been because my father died four months prior. That afternoon, she asked me if I would come see her when she died. She wanted to make sure I would go to the cemetery. She had understood what a cemetery was. She also asked if her boys were dead. She remembered she had sons, but didn't know if they were alive. She couldn't remember their names and she didn't remember she had three daughters.

These questions lasted all afternoon. I couldn't get her mind off her boys. She complained that she wasn't a good mother if her boys were alive and they didn't visit with her. I was saddened by these words. I told her many times that she was the best mother in the world, but she never believed me. This conversation was repeated continually.

As I sat beside her bed in the evening, I told her how much her children love her. I told her to shut her eyes and rest. I rubbed noses with her as I did every night. She asked me why I called her "Mom" because she only had boys. I couldn't answer her without crying. I couldn't understand why the disease allowed her to remember her sons who didn't visit much, but wouldn't let her remember me who took care of her every day. After a few minutes, I told my mother that she was the mother I had always wanted. She didn't understand me but smiled anyway. I felt relieved. I could go to sleep because she smiled.

Besides me, my mother had two other daughters. She never talked about them, either, which brought me a little comfort, because at least it wasn't just *me* she was forgetting. As I stood outside her door to make sure she didn't leave her bed, I thought about the smile and hoped her eyes would stay shut long enough for her to sleep.

I could tell by her breathing if she was asleep or not. I hurried to shower and got ready for bed, because I knew when my eyes shut I would be in a deep sleep. I couldn't sleep until I was certain my mother was asleep. I got worried that my mother would wake and wander the house and that I wouldn't hear her. I told my husband about my mother's smile and that made it a good day. Most nights, my husband would ask me, after I was ready for bed, how things went that day. Talking in bed was the only time we had. He lost a lot of sleep because he loved his mother-in-law dearly.

Trouble with Words

Although my mother was in an unusual good mood, her words made no sense, and she knew it. I felt sorry for her. After a few attempts to talk, and the right words wouldn't come, she said, "Shoot! I shut up." I laughed so hard that it even made her laugh.

Not only did her words not come out right, but also she jumped from one subject to another more than normal. She talked about her two boys. Then she would say she needed butter on her gown. Then she would mention her purse, and we would begin the search for it by tearing apart her room. She didn't find it and stayed in her room looking for it. She never got upset. When I told my husband that she was in her room looking for her purse, he became worried. I explained that my mother was in a good mood all day. He went to her room and couldn't believe that she smiled. She tried to talk to him but had trouble with her words so he left her to search for her purse.

Later, she came into the family room and sat in her gold chair. I realized that this was the quietest day I had since my mother moved in our house. It was the only one. After that day, my mother began to talk less and less. From then on, my mother had trouble with her words. She would mean one thing but say something else. Sometimes, she noticed it. Other times, she didn't. It embarrassed her, so we acted like we didn't notice. We realized that even though she had no memory, her feelings were sensitive. We wanted to treat her with the respect she deserved in her later years and especially with her illness.

Reversal of Roles

Funny, it seemed as if the roles of parenthood had been reversed as I hid behind the door and watched my mother go back to her room. She was hurrying, and quite pleased with herself, with two cookies in her hand. She thought she had snuck them from the kitchen, even though I had placed them on the counter for her. She didn't eat much at dinner that night so I knew she would be hungry and also knew she wouldn't ask for food.

As she hurried down the hall, I smile at her in her purple gown, which was all faded and worn. The only one she wore. She had gotten new ones, but she went back to the dirty clothes to get the purple one, or she changed back into her clothes and slept in her clothes, rather than "someone else's" gown. The other gowns belonged to someone else. She said she wouldn't wear someone else's clothes.

Her thick legs showed, because the gown had shrunk so much over the years. I smiled at her thick legs. She was as a child getting up for the 10th time to get a drink. I had to keep reminding myself she was my mother, and I loved her so much. I wondered, if she were living somewhere else, if she would go to bed hungry.

I thought about the purple gown. My daughter and I had spent every spare minute, for a week, shopping for another purple gown that looked similar to the one she wore. This night, a friend told me she saw a purple gown in another town. I guess everyone we knew was looking for a purple gown for my mother. I made the trip to go look at it and bought it. She now had two purple gowns, the new one that I bleached to make it look old and the old one. She also had one purple robe with sleeves torn out of the back of one arm.

Every few days, my husband asked me if I could sew the arm on my mother's robe. I told him it couldn't be repaired and that it had shrunk. It was too small for her, but she recognized it and wouldn't put on another one. I found it like fighting with a child over their security blanket. Of course, I also fought with my mother over a blanket. She took all the blankets from her room except two and had put them in the hallway or another bedroom. This continued for weeks. They weren't hers, she said, even though we moved them from her house. After awhile I put them into the hall closet, except the two that were acceptable. They stayed out folded on her sofa.

I left my hiding place to go to her room. I went to see if she was in bed. I carried a glass of water with me, in case she was thirsty. As I peeked into her room, I saw her put a tissue in her purse to hide. I asked her what she was doing. She said, "Oh. Don't tell anyone, but I snuck out some food. You never know when you'll get to eat again." She offered me a bite. I told her to hide it for tomorrow. She put it in her purse and put her purse in her trunk. She said she was thirsty because the owners didn't have a sink in the place. I gave her the glass of water, but she said it belonged to someone else. It had "germs". I finally convinced her that I had been looking for her with the glass of water; that it was a clean glass. It was strange that my mother couldn't remember me, but could remember about germs.

The difference between a child and an Alzheimer's patient is trust. Children trust everyone, especially their parents. Alzheimer's patients don't trust anyone. But as the disease worsened, she trusted me more. Even though she didn't know who I was, if I was in the room with three other people, she would come over to me and stand near me like she needed protection. She also whispered to me so no one else could hear her. That made me want to protect her even more.

At that point, even though I was tired of talking and walking, I wasn't upset with her. She still made a good argument, like the germs on a glass of water. I was so glad she was able to get around the house by herself, although I could see that she was slowing down rapidly.

The Special Clothes

A care worker, from the insurance company, came by one afternoon to fill out paper work for my mother's insurance. She asked for a list of medicines that my mother took daily. I told her a "good night" pill every other night. The worker couldn't believe it. She said, "This lady is 86 years old and doesn't take a dozen pills a day, that's great." My mother looked at her and said, "I know I'm old. Jesus is my doctor and always has been." We both looked at mom smiling. We said, "Sounds like a great doctor.

Maybe, we should try him." My mother seemed pleased and was nice to the insurance worker after that.

Later that evening, my mother took off her green sweater and handed it to me. She said, "Here, you can give this back to whomever it belongs to." I didn't want to tell her it was her favorite sweater. I was saddened because my mother was so kind about wanting to return it to its owner.

The next morning, my mother left her room very early, already dressed. She didn't wait for me to lay out her clothes. She had on her favorite yellow cotton pants and white T-shirt with a yellow flower on it. It was funny because they were brand new clothes to her. She asked if she could keep the clothes, because they looked good on her, and fit her just right. I told her the owners left the clothes so she could wear them. She was so excited to be wearing new clothes that fit. I smiled because she had worn them the day before, and I had just washed them last night, and hung them back up in her closet.

It turned out to be a good day. She paced a lot, but she wasn't angry. Later, in the evening, my mother was worried about her husband being able to find her. She kept saying, "Will he know where I am? Does he know how to get here?" We assured her he did know where she was and how to get there. We had hoped this would stop her worrying, but it continued throughout the night. Then, she worried about Alfred's two friends who got him into trouble. She also worried about Alfred's truck that constantly broke down. My husband told her Alfred would be at the house later, but stopped to spend the night at David's house. David was my brother. We hoped she would remember him, but she didn't so we said he was Alfred's friend. She immediately assumed he was the no good friend that she didn't like. That started my mother on her tirade again. My husband decided to leave, since he no longer had any ideas. He said, "Linda will tell you where Alfred is."

Then, my mother told me she knew a Linda who was a baby and wondered what had happened to her. I had to talk about myself as if I wasn't in the room. That was hard for me. But at least we had gotten off the subject of where Alfred was.

Chapter 7
No Regrets

As I thought about my experience with my mother, it struck me instantly. I didn't have any regrets. I decided that had to be the name of a chapter in this book. I have realized that I have so much joy from caring for my mother, those last few years. I can't think of one event, or activity, in two years that made as much a difference on my life as caring for her did. I believe caregivers arrive at a point when they don't regret the choices they make to help a loved one.

Peace of Mind

There is a delicate balance to share work with family care. Although I was fortunate enough to bring home my work, not all Alzheimer's caregivers have that option.

Caring for my mother gave me peace of mind and a new strength to handle the problems of life. I learned that the things in life I missed became of little value compared to caring for her. The grandchildren would have other birthday parties. I would have other opportunities to attend church services. Saturday night dinners, out with my husband and friends, are being enjoyed now. All my true friends say they missed me during those few years, but caring for my mother didn't make a difference in our relationship or friendship.

I want to let all caregivers, who read this book, to know the task is daunting, but it's rewarding. People can care for a loved one themselves, and they should feel compelled to do so.

Someday, I hope there will be more education on Alzheimer's. I hope there will be more books to read, and more modern medicine available. I hope doctors will be able to test early for the disease and begin treatment early. I hope we won't be discussing the disease in a whisper, but out loud so all can understand, and not be embarrassed by it.

When people love patients enough, and finally connect with them and their disease, they find it becomes easier to care for them. They are seen as they really are at this stage in life; like a young child. I believe that talking to them like a child, with love and patience, will lead to no regrets for caregivers. Jesus said, "Let the children come." In this case, it was my elderly mother, who was a child, in her mind.

Care Homes

My daughter and I set out to check into a long-term care facility for my mother. After visiting three, I thought my mother could stay with us a little longer. I'm sure the facilities did the best job they could, but it wasn't for us.

My mother started her usual pacing at 4:30 p.m. She walked back and forth through the house asking, "Where am I going to live? Who can take me home?" Wringing her hands, I could tell that she needed reassurance and she would be safe. Fear had already set in her mind. The experts call the symptoms, "sun downers."

I wondered if I would have made the same decision, if I had went looking at care facilities at 4:30 p.m., when she started pacing. Just then, my husband came into the kitchen and asked, "Did you get a chance to go see a few places?" He carefully avoided saying "care homes" in front of my mother. I looked at him with tears in my eyes.

"Is it OK if she stays here for right now? I'm sure we can do a much better job caring for her than strangers."

My husband said, "You know I love her and fear for her safety just as much as you do. Her mind has been misplaced with Alzheimer's. There is nothing that can change that."

But he understood that I needed to know someone was caring for my mother. I understood what he meant. I knew there was not a thing in the world I could do about her being misplaced. I only could protect her physically, by being in close contact. I needed her in my house for my own peace of mind.

My daughter said, "Mom, why move Grandma? If you did, you would be living at the care facility making sure she was safe. You should care for her at your home as long as you can."

We tried to comfort my mother, hugging her to let her know there was nothing to fear in this house. We stayed up with her, as long as she needed to be reassured, before she fell asleep. My mother was afraid the doors weren't locked. She had to turn on the lights to make sure the house was safe. She didn't take our word for it. That night, she went from room to room checking everything and made sure all outside doors were locked.

Despite all of this, I was sure I had made the right decision to keep my mother with us. If she were in a care facility, she would have been afraid of everything outside her room. I couldn't rest easy that night because I was worried about her. Night time was the worst for my mother.

So we took it one day, and one night, at a time. I decided to care for her as long as I could. I knew she would have done the same for me.

It saddens me to go into care homes and see the caregivers making fun of Alzheimer's patients, which my daughter and I saw, or not paying attention to them. I also felt angry when I heard family members wouldn't visit their loved ones because they were labeled as bitter, mean old people. I know they aren't. In my mother's case, her world would become wrapped up in a twisted rolled up paper towel, a scrap of food, and a bed for sleeping.

Preparing for Eternity

I feel so fortunate and blessed to have helped to care for my aging mother for the last two years. My father died after carrying the burden for five years. His wish was that my mother not be placed in a care facility. I honored that wish.

My mother was getting well-deserved care from my family then. My mother had many grandchildren and great grandchildren. A few years ago, she had remembered all of their names. She used to bake them their favorite desserts every time they visited. She remembered their birthdays and Christmas, before she forgot there was a Christmas. She bought every stocking that K Mart had. With my sister, we wrapped all of the little gifts she had. She said, "No child in this family will be without a gift."

When I got so tired and my body wanted to fail me, I thought, "I can't miss one minute with my mother." She deserves the best care in the world. I motivated myself by thinking this was a short play that would soon be over. Act II would come soon enough.

After she had exited the stage, I would be able to keep going and return to my normal life.

Still, I had to consider my purpose in this short play. I begin reading a popular inspirational book and realized I had a purpose. I was preparing for eternity by caring for my 88-year-old mother. I love her and couldn't manage my life without her. I reflected on how she cared for my six siblings and me. She devoted her whole life to us.

There certainly were many times I would think or tell my husband I couldn't do the work the next day. He would say, "Wait for tomorrow. Then see if you can say that."

My daughter or niece could tell when I was at that point, and many times, came to my rescue by saying, "I'll stay with Grandma tonight for a few hours. You go out to dinner." Before dinner was over, though, I felt the urge to call home, or just go home to see how my mother was. My mind had become a time clock. My mother used to say, "Whatever you do here on Earth will come back to you. It will also prepare you for eternity."

Chapter 8
Second Period of Adjustment

Just as caregivers need a time to adjust to having an Alzheimer's patient live with them, they also must take time after the person dies, or goes into a care facility, to readjust. There is no down time while caring for the patient. It takes every waking moment of every day to care for and prepare for the needs of the patient. When that ends, caregivers have a tendency to rush to the kitchen or bedroom to see why they don't hear any noises or why no one is yelling for help. Then, they realize the person is gone, which leaves an empty feeling inside the caregivers.

After Death

The second night, after my mother passed away, I was asleep. I felt a tight grip on my upper arm. My mother stood beside the bed with her hand on my arm.

She said softly, "Linda." She squeezed my arm and said, "Linda" again. I reached over to grab her hand still feeling the pressure on my arm. I tried to sit up in bed. I said, "What Mom? Is everything OK? Can't you sleep tonight?"

As I talked to her in the dark, I realized she couldn't have been standing there, because she was dead, and in heaven. My husband woke up and asked what was happening. He said, "Who are you talking to? Are you OK?"

I told him, "Mom was here beside my bed. She said two words –Linda. Linda–and squeezed my arm. I felt it. She was here."

My husband said, "At least, she remembered your name. Try to go back to sleep." He was trying to add some humor to the situation.

I will never forget that moment. I can still hear it today. I guess it was her way of letting me know she remembered me, and my name. The squeeze on the arm was to tell me she loved me.

A Quiet House

It was the day after my mother's funeral. I noticed that my mother's dog was gone. The first few nights, after my mother died, the dog would come to my bedroom at night and lay on the floor on my side of the bed. We had a lot of company from out of town and had a full house, so I didn't notice the dog was gone right away. I asked my husband about the dog. I wasn't worried because I still had a few people in the house to feed and other dogs.

My husband said my family had put the dog into my brother's car that evening, after my mother's service. He said the dog would be living with my brother. I was angry and shocked. Even though I wasn't a big dog person, and at first, didn't like the dog, I felt like I lost my mother and dog at the same time. I was concerned that my mother would be upset if she knew I wasn't taking care of her dog.

My husband and brother told me that it was a hard thing to do, but it was a necessary thing to be done, the way they did. My brother knew he would be caring for the dog eventually. My father had requested that he care for the dog, before his death. I knew that.

Without the jingling of the dog tags and my mother asking where to find the bathroom, I found the house too quiet. My mother depended on me for a lot. After her death, I didn't have to rush. I wasn't in a hurry anymore, but it took me a long time to remember that. I wasn't able to slow down at first. I would still call home every morning to see how things were going. I said "no" to people when they asked me to do extra work or volunteer at the church. I just answered that I had to be at home.

One day, my daughter called to ask me to lunch. I told her I had to be home in 30 minutes. She said, "Mom, you can do whatever you want now, anytime you want." I said, "Yes I can." It was still hard to adjust to the quiet house. I knew I had to handle my mother's affairs, and take care of bank accounts, and go through her belongings. I realized I had gotten so attached to caring for my mother, that the time after her death wasn't any different. I never noticed that she wasn't there in her body any more. She had left long ago in her mind.

Since that first week after she died, I have seen the dog a few times a year. She is having fun running around on a big farm in the country, with three other dogs.

Cleaning Closets

Over the next year, I cleaned the hall closet or bathroom shelves. As I did these tasks, I would find a rolled up tissue or paper towel stuck in the back. I found some in the cracks of the bottom drawers. She either had food, at one time hidden in those places for the dog, or just little pieces of paper that belonged to her were hidden. Each time, I came across something that she did or something that reminded me of her, I cried. I still cry. I still think about how small her world became.

The Candle

In October, after my mother died, I put out the Halloween decorations. I remembered a white glass candle my children gave me that I wasn't able to use before.

Every time I put the candle on the coffee table, my mother thought it was a glass of milk. She would repeat over and over that someone had left a glass of milk in the living room and claimed it would spill. After a few days of moving the candle from table to kitchen and back again, my husband said to put away the candle. It saved me steps and gave me a little peace of mind. I was a little resentful, but I also found it amusing. After a while, the constant moving of the candle got old.

I didn't take out that candle again, for more than a year after she passed away. We smiled as we relived the story again. I missed her. She came up with things that were funny, strange, interesting and aggravating all at the same time. Her time, with my husband and I, changed our lives and put our lives on hold, but we have so many memories.

My Most Valuable Person

They say that time heals. It has been more than a year since my mother died and I think back to the last few months of my mothers' life. It's as almost as if time hurt. Seeing what she was going through didn't make any sense to me because of who she was and how she lived her life.

Recently, I was at a Bible study class. When a question was asked about who we thought was the most important person of value in our lives, I thought of her even though she has been gone for a year. The hurt came back, almost as if she were still here.

As each one in the room answered the question, I answered my mother, but didn't give her name. At that moment, I was overcome with emotion not just because of what a good person she was but mostly how unfair her last few years has been to her, because of Alzheimer's disease.

I thought about it all the way home at how my mother was the biggest influence in my life. She taught me my principles, my morals, and standards. She didn't just teach them to me; she showed them as well, by living them herself.

I can always reflect that my mother taught me to be honest and do good to others. "That's what you want a return on in your life," she would say.

And so it seems so strange that someone who did nothing but good, her whole life, lived her last few years very sad, very unhappy and very angry at everyone around her.

And just one day after I said that my mother was the biggest influence of good in my life, my eight-year-old granddaughter asked me, "Grandma, do you know what you will name a book about Grandma Ruby? A book has to have a name you know" as if she was giving me information I needed to know.

Of course I had the name long before I started the book, "Why Do You Call Me Mom?" She looked at me and said, "Oh Yes. Grandma Ruby forgot that you were her daughter," and as she said that, with a sad frown on her face I got all choked up again trying not to let her see my tears. We sat and talked about Grandma Ruby, not remembering anyone or anything and how she acted like a kid, sometimes herself, and that there is a name for the illness that makes old people act as they cannot help it. As she went outside to play, I thought that even now, after a year that she passed away, I have this horrible sick feeling in my stomach of when my mother would turn around and look at me so puzzled and say after I called her mom.

"Why do you call me Mom?"

This woman, who had high integrity and was so precious, within the life of her family and friends didn't even know I was her daughter, much less know she had seven children who loved her very much. It seemed strange that this book contained a small portion of her life that I kept in a journal. That's not the person she was. I don't know how I can write a book on such a small portion of her life lasting for only a few years where I documented the actions that were the opposite of who that person was.

All of my mother's good deeds won't be written. I only wrote about the problems she caused us. That makes me sad. I want the world to know who my mother was. She was active and healthy, and was the kindest parent and grandparent there ever could be. She wasn't what's in this book.

As I write this, it sounds like a selfish feeling within me, but it's not totally selfish. It is a feeling of sadness for me, and a feeling that I must protect her who doesn't know her own daughter, if that makes sense.

Now, it is my turn in protecting the one who taught me all that is good, and that what I did by caring for her is good, even if she didn't know I was her daughter and I had to put on hold two years of my life to take care of her.

This disease robbed my mother of her personality, not just her memory, but also her joy. It made her become someone she wasn't. Isn't it so strange that there are medicines for depression, personality changes and other mental illnesses? There are anger management classes for angry people. These people can take a pill or a class and get up the next day feeling more like themselves and half way back to normal, a better person, even than they were yesterday.

But people with Alzheimer's have to experience constant change. If there is one thing to be thankful for, it is that they don't know it. But all the loved ones around them and caregivers know it. We are the ones to feel sadness for them. Maybe there should be a medicine for us.

It is so important to get the word around, somehow, that Alzheimer's patients cannot, and should not be held responsible for the way they act or what they say. They need to be in an environment that doesn't affect a lot of people, emotionally, or that holds them responsible for their memory loss.

I found out quickly that nearly all people do not deal well with rejection, and that's what it's like to be around an Alzheimer's patient. Early in the morning, I would remind myself from the first "Good Morning, Mom" through the end of the day that I have now entered into her world. It's the same world I live in for today. I have the ability to jump back into my world, although she would never be able to join me in mine again, so I had to join her as she regressed and went back, way back to an earlier age and younger years; of which now from what the doctor said is about 11 years old. But, at times, acts much younger.

My mother cared for me with great joy and a sense of pride, from what my aunts tell me. I had the pleasure of repaying my mother, by attending to her needs and protecting her from those who did not understand Alzheimer's, who thought that tomorrow she would wake up and remember everyone and join them in their world.

If it could only be that way, but it cannot. They shouldn't be held responsible. It is a disease that is beyond their means. It is irreversible. But there is so much we can do to make their life more comfortable, with a feeling of safety. My purpose soon became only to make my mother feel safe and to have some food out on the counter at all times, so she knew she would not go hungry. Feeling safe and full was all she ever talked about, or showed emotions about. Even the food issue became less and less as the disease worsened.

Enjoying the Family Again

Since her death, I have been thinking that I might someday lose my memory like my mother did. My children and I talk about it some, but for now, we are finally catching up and enjoying each other again. I probably do think about Alzheimer's more than they do, or they don't tell me if they are thinking about it now. I watch television in the evenings. I can see the news all the way through the broadcast without any interruptions. I'm cooking out on the grill again. I have the knobs back on my stove. I have all my clothes hanging in my closet again. I'm excited to hear about the new research, and new medications available for Alzheimer's disease now. My hope is that just as much time and money will be spent teaching caregivers. They need to learn so much if they are to be successful. As we accept this disease into our generation, we must open up and talk about our experiences. It will help improve the care of the patient, and provide the caregivers with more information on what to do.

This is my story only, and from my point of view, taken from a two-year journal. There are many other stories that I didn't write in this book that fill the pages of two journals. My family read from the original journal when they come to visit, almost as much as they go through the family photo album. My grandchildren have better memories of their great-grandmother. They accepted her disease for what it was and tried only to remember her kinder years. When we talked about her illness, it helped them to understand it.

Remembering Mom

As I wrote in my journal, every evening or early morning, it never entered my mind that I would be writing it again, only in book form this time. And now, as I write this book, I will face family members who will cheer me to continue, and others who will say, "Put Mother to rest. Don't let others know what we went through," thinking this is more of a mental illness that we need to hide. Nonetheless, others will go through the very same thing, day after day and year after year. I think it's important to talk about Alzheimer's. We need to be able to say, out loud, "my mother has Alzheimer's," so the person told will understand it just as clearly as if we said, "my mother has heart disease."

I, in my mind, sometimes challenge the notion that experts believe Alzheimer's develops because of one not using their mental ability and/or becoming inactive physically. Because in Mother's case, she was so very active, tending one of the largest gardens in her small town. She cooked by memory, which was amazing. However, it turned out to be dire in the end, because now we have no written documentation of her recipes to keep in the family. Until Dad pulled the plug, and told her the treadmill was broken because he was worried about her balance, she still walked on it for thirty minutes every morning. She also walked around the neighborhood every evening after dinner. She loved to read books, mostly the Bible; and we called her "the Newscaster" because she read the newspaper daily and quoted from it. She would tear out the pages from mail order magazines to order seeds for her garden, and also show Dad his next new project that he could construct out of wood.

My dad said he knew early on when she became less interested in all of their yard projects; and even much less interested in talking to their neighbors and not wanting to speak to the family by phone. I only know, that in my mother's case, she stopped living *after* Alzheimer's took over, not before. And for that, I can be grateful and proud of all of her accomplishments and the good memories she has left my family and me.